living with
your *imperfect*
back

by Lori Heimann
& Jane Taylor

who live with imperfect backs

Your Imperfect Back

By Lori Heimann & Jane Taylor

Published by IngramSpark

International Standard Book Number 979-8-9892695-0-1

Printed in the United States of America

Edited by Dawn Ronco, *DawnRonco.com*

Illustrations by Scott Fray, *LivingBrush.com*

www.imperfectback.com

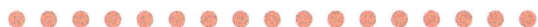

feedback from readers

From Doctors & Medical Professionals

I have known Jane and Lori for many years. Both ladies have taken control of their symptoms and their lives, and they have become powerful and resourceful advocates over the years. Even though they still navigate their pain daily, they lead full and interactive lives. I see this book as the next step in their process to help others who can benefit from what they have learned on their journeys. I think it will fill a much-needed void.

Lorraine Kingham, PT, MTC, CMTPT, *BritPT.com*

This is very valuable information for patients with back pain issues!

Dr. Wesley Ibazebo, Physiatrist, *MurphyWainer.com*

A book that reads like a conversation with a friend. It's a wealth of knowledge for anyone who struggles with back pain.

Kelsey Crews, LMBT

feedback from readers

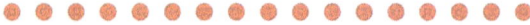

● ● ● ● ● ● ● ● ● ● ● ● ● ● ● ● ●

I have known Lori for a good part of her back pain and surgeries. Having a handbook from a patient's perspective such as Lori's will benefit so many people. I endorse this handbook based on its detailed descriptions of covering all the bases that an individual will face and deal with chronic back and surgical conditions.

> Dr. John O'Halloran, Owner, *OHalloranRehabilitation.com*

I am so impressed with this book! I'm a very critical reader, and I found this book to be well considered, thorough and easy to follow. I am sure it will be a blessing to many people. Thank you, Jane and Lori, for putting the time and effort into helping others who are living with back pain.

> Maggie Keskinen, Pilates Instructor

Jane is a long-term patient, and we think that what she and Lori are doing with this book is GREAT! We see patients on both ends of their surgical journey, staving off surgery for years or helping patients' post-surgery return to wellness. This book shows what the road ahead can look like for anyone with back problems. There are many people out there who are ready to help you.

> Dr. Tim Clark & Dr. Dean Meylor, *MeylorChiropractic.org*

From Other Back Pain Patients

The book gave me fresh ideas. I am supposed to have surgery soon. My lower back fusion has failed so I must fuse to another level. We must roll with the punches and get on with life like Jane says. Hope everyone enjoys the book as much as I have and takes its suggestions for a better life.

> Nancy Rowsey, NC

● ● ● ● ● ● ● ● ● ● ● ● ● ● ● ● ● ● ●

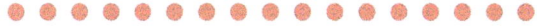

I have inoperable back problems. Lori and Jane's advice has been a game-changer in helping me control my pain so that my life is livable again. I'm forever grateful to them!

    Lois Slove Losyk, NC

I so appreciate all the personal notes and insights from Jane and Lori! If you have back pain, I definitely recommend reading their thoughtful ideas so you can benefit from their experience.

    Bobbie Matela, NC

Your book is terrific! It comfortably addresses almost all the questions and fears that folks enduring back pain experience in understandable, reassuring, layman terms. I can see this being offered as a resource by back surgeons and even physical therapists for their patients. I wish it was available when I was going through my back issues. Well done!

    Barry Leibowitz, GA

This book is very well organized and is an easy-to-understand compilation of "DIY" advice for getting your back fixed and keeping it fixed. Back problems are challenging in the best of circumstances, and this book offers an exceptional resource for anyone who is contemplating both surgical and non-surgical solutions. I truly wish this book had been available 20 years ago before I faced serious back problems! I have personally "been there, done that" and recommend this book to all who face similar issues.

    Gary Brown, NC

terms to know about your back

Your back is made up of bones, discs, and nerves.

In your spine are 33 bones, called vertebrae.

- The top 8 are grouped as "cervical" or neck.
- The middle 12 are "thoracic" or mid-back.
- The bottom 5 are "lumbar" or low-back.
- The sacrum is 1 large fused bone below lumbar and is the back part of your pelvis.
- Coccyx is the very bottom, your "tail bone."

In between the vertebrae are discs, squishy cushions that allow the bones to move and flex as needed.

Your spinal column runs from your brain through the middle of your vertebrae. It regulates movement, distributes nerves throughout your body, and controls reflexes.

Below are some problems that can arise with your discs and vertebrae:

Cervical Spine Vertebrae

Thoracic Spine Vertebrae

Lumbar Spine Vertebrae

Sacrum

Coccyx

C1
C2
C3
C4
C5
C6
C7
C8
T1
T2
T3
T4
T5
T6
T7
T8
T9
T10
T11
T12
L1
L2
L3
L4
L5
S1
S2
S3
S4
S5

NORMAL INTERVERTEBRAL DISC

DEGENERATED DISC

BULGING DISC

THINNING DISC

HERNIATED DISC

DISC DEGENERATION WITH OSTEOPHYTE FORMATION

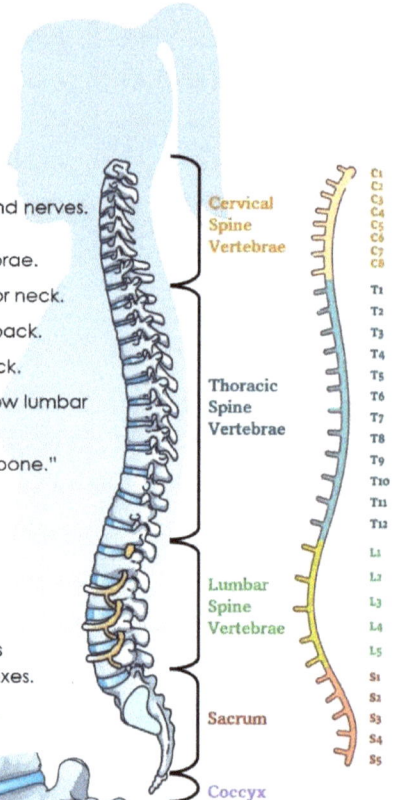

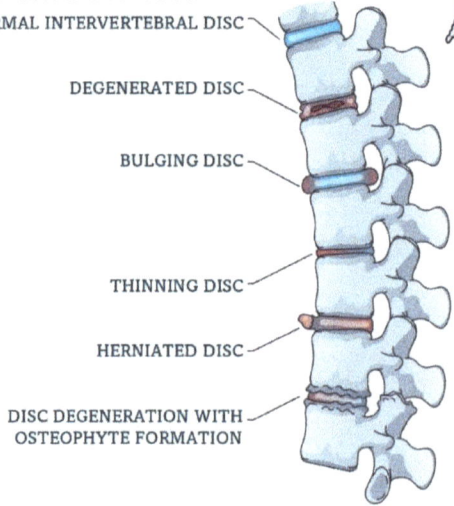

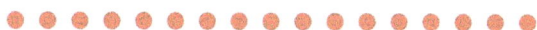

table
of
contents

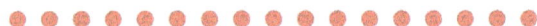

who wrote this?

What makes us qualified to write a book about back pain? We're spinal surgery patients, and this book comes from our experiences living with our own imperfect backs. We've done a great deal of research about backs and back pain. We've learned from our doctors and other medical professionals we've worked with over the years. We think our stories can convince you that a good life is still possible, even with an imperfect back!

LORI

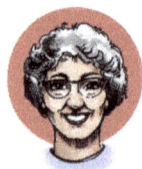

My back troubles started in 1994, and my first neurologist said fusion surgery wasn't necessary. Throughout the years from 1994 until 2006, I saw quite a few doctors and none of them had a solution for my pain, until I found Dr. Mark Roy. Dr. Roy is a smart, skilled neurosurgeon who showed particular compassion. He was never too busy to listen and explain things to me. He diagnosed me with degenerative disc disease, spinal stenosis, and severe sciatica. He performed my first spinal fusion in 2007. While the fusion reduced the pain, I still suffered.

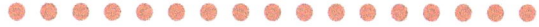

In 2009, I had a spinal stimulator implanted. It helped for two years, but ultimately didn't solve my pain.

In early 2011, I fell while working and fractured my T12. This required my second operation, which was essentially a T11-L1 lateral fusion.

In 2013, I was diagnosed with "flat back," which is a condition in which the lower spine loses some of its normal curvature. I underwent another surgery for this and two days later had an additional operation for a thoracic spine fracture. That fused me from T11-S1. I developed "gluteal amnesia" or "dead butt syndrome" – where the gluteus medius stops working.

For months following each surgery, I wore a back brace and restricted my motions such as bending, lifting, and twisting. I continue with physical therapy to this day to help maintain my strength, mobility, and flexibility. I consciously have to think about what I'm doing in order to take care of myself. I don't want to overdo it.

*I haven't stopped doing the things I love;
I just change the way I do them.*

In 2019, I was fused from T8-L1. That was my last surgery, as well as the most difficult and painful. Unfortunately, as a result I developed Trendelenburg gait. After so many surgeries, doctors' appointments, physical therapy appointments, and battery replacements for my implant, I still struggle with pain and mobility. The surgeries corrected anatomical problems and were necessary, but they didn't "fix" me. My current diagnosis is Adult Degenerative Scoliosis, which affects my posture, my gait, and my self-esteem. I wish my back functioned well, but I'm living with what I have.

who wrote this?

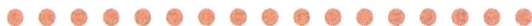

● ● ● ● ● ● ● ● ● ● ● ● ● ● ● ● ● ●

I've always looked after other people. I continue my volunteer work, despite the pain in my back, because it gives me joy. I'm a very giving, loving, and caring person with grit and determination.

Through this book, my mission is to help educate you in ways to get better, move better, and feel better.

JANE

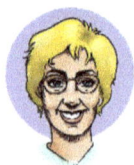

I experienced my first severe back pain when I was 19 years old and in college. It took a whole year to try to fix it... with no improvement. I finally went to Duke Hospital for a spinal fusion of the L5-S1.

From my point of view, the reason for surgery is to relieve pain so that I can get on with my life.

The good news is that the fusion worked. It relieved my pain, and after recuperating for about five months, I went back to college. As time went on, I learned to keep my weight down and to exercise consistently to keep my back happy.

Decades later, I experienced a muscle spasm in my back that didn't release for months. *Oh, no... here we go again!* This time, there was no surgical means of correction. So, I've explored a bunch of alternatives, and a combination of treatments are keeping me active.

Now I focus on pain relief through multiple approaches: the pain management office, gentle exercise in the pool at my local YMCA, regular chiropractic care, relaxation through massage, physical therapy, gratitude, and mindfulness. Rest and quality sleep have become central for my health.

● ● ● ● ● ● ● ● ● ● ● ● ● ● ● ● ● ● ●

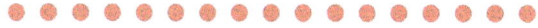

I currently teach water exercise classes at my local YMCA, sharing my knowledge with other people who live with pain.

I've discovered that I understand people in pain in a way that I never did before. A person who hasn't experienced pain cannot truly empathize.

It's become a blessing to share our common experiences and to encourage those who are still living with debilitating pain.

FROM BOTH OF US

Your Body is Unique

We can tell you how we take care of ourselves, but we can't tell you exactly how it will work out for you. Ultimately, you must be your own advocate. Since you live in your body, you're the one to take care of it. While anatomy and body chemistry are similar in all humans, no one's body is exactly like someone else's. What works for one person may not work for another. If a treatment works for you, woohoo! If it doesn't, just move on and try something else.

*Pain can be depressing.
Pain can take away our self-confidence
and our feisty spirits.
Pain can make us cry.
We can only do our best as we live
this beautiful, blessed life.*

People often ask us, "How can you be so cheerful when you're living in such pain?" Our answer is the same: "Because we choose to."

who wrote this?

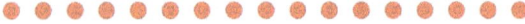

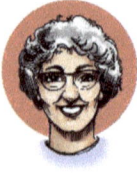

● ● ● ● ● ● ● ● ● ● ● ● ● ● ● ● ●

I've tried to not let my pain define who and what I am. This pain and "dead butt" causes trouble with my balance and makes it difficult to walk any distance. But I won't let it prevent me from doing what I want to do. Some days are hard and others are harder, but I choose to work through the pain. I'm not a martyr, I'm just doing the best I can with what I have. As I look back over the years, I feel substantially better than I did, I have less pain, and I'm grateful and blessed for the life I get to live.

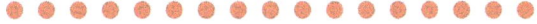

At age 19, I was lying in a hospital bed, and I couldn't reach the blanket at the foot of the bed. That was when I really understood that my life had drastically changed. At that moment, I realized that I had a choice — and I continue to make this choice every day:

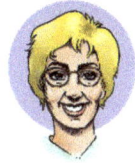

I can be miserable. I can wallow in negative thoughts and self-pity, I can be angry over how unfair life is, and I can make people around me miserable, too...

OR

I can choose to be mostly happy. I can discipline my thoughts to stay away from long deliberation over my pain and the changes it requires. I can choose to see the positive aspects of life, especially when they arise out of troubled times. I'm not always successful, but my life is better when I'm optimistic.

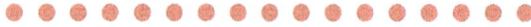

fore-word & back-word

We're indebted to our advisors and contributors, Dr. Mark Roy and Dr. Joseph Stern. These esteemed neurosurgeons lent a combined 60 years of medical expertise, and their kindness and compassion have made them outstanding doctors.

FORE-WORD

Mark Roy, M.D., Ph.D., Neurosurgeon
Lori's Spine Surgeon

When Lori asked me to look at the book she was writing with Jane, she had been my patient for over 20 years. I realized that in most of her back adventures, I had been a willing participant.

I was pleasantly surprised that this work is not a technical treatise on spine surgery but an invaluable how-to guide for patients with chronic and acute back pain, both surgical and nonsurgical.

Hard science is invaluable and cannot be discounted. But Lori and Jane's journey reminds us it is the individual patient's perception of the care we render and our interactions with them that ultimately determine success or failure in the surgical sphere.

● ● ● ● ● ● ● ● ● ● ● ● ● ● ● ● ●

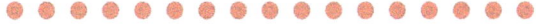

This work relates 50 cumulative years of back pain management experience of Lori and Jane. It provides valuable recommendations and insights for other individuals with disabling back pain.

BACK-WORD

Dr. Joseph Stern, Neurosurgeon, Author, Inventor
JosephSternMD.com

I am honored to provide a backstop to Lori and Jane's account of being patients and reluctant travelers in the world of spinal surgery. They are lending suggestions to other patients based on wisdom gained through their own challenges and experiences.

Lori and Jane offer practical information, but mostly they give reassurance: these things you're feeling are common; we've been through them, too. Your pain is likely to get better or certainly become more tolerable. You are not alone. We will help you cope and show you how. What a gift of themselves these ladies have given to you!

I have recently become a surgical patient myself, and I'm having to adjust to new limitations and expectations. While back pain doesn't usually kill you, living in pain can rob you of your vitality. Losing capabilities you have taken for granted can be scary, isolating, and depressing. Having someone hold your hand and guide you with their hard-won wisdom is a gift and can make all the difference.

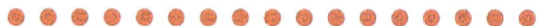

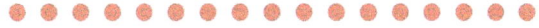

finding answers to your pain

DOES THIS SOUND FAMILIAR TO YOU?

- Getting up in the morning is now ridiculously difficult for me because my back hurts.
- I often have to stop to rest my back.
- My back prevents me from doing the things I did before.
- When my doctor says "get some exercise," I laugh because exercise makes my pain worse.
- I have to turn down some fun invitations because I hurt too much.
- My pain is intense. I feel it every day. It interferes with the things I love and the activities I used to take for granted. It wears me out.

If you think any of these things, this book is for you. Your life has already been changed by back pain. We understand. We've been there.

Whether your back aches sometimes, or flares up when you work too hard, or keeps you from living your best life, this book is for you. Living with back pain forces us to "listen" to our bodies. Sometimes, our backs are so upset that they clamp down with

● ● ● ● ● ● ● ● ● ● ● ● ● ● ● ● ●

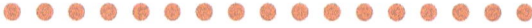

pain, forcing us to stop whatever we're doing. This is pain that we can't just push through. This is pain that interrupts our lives. Now, our bodies have our attention.

It's hard to know what to do, especially when the pain interferes with regular life and clear thinking. You may be considering surgery. You may be wondering what else is possible. This book will take you through what we've learned. Sometimes surgery is the right answer, but the majority of people with back pain don't need surgery. You can find out your own solutions.

It's time for you to take charge of your own health. After all, no one knows your body like you do. No one can say if the pain is getting better or worse, except you. Therefore, you'll make decisions that are best for your own body.

We're back patients like you, and we're offering you practical ways to live with your imperfect back. You and your doctor will decide whether surgery is right for you. This book encourages you to make the best decisions for yourself and provides help with whatever you decide. We share experiences from our real lives, living with spinal fusion and our own imperfect backs.

FIND GREAT MEDICAL PROFESSIONALS

First, you need wonderful medical professionals to work with. We encourage you to meet doctors, surgeons, neurologists, orthopedists, pain specialists, physical therapists, massage therapists, chiropractors, acupuncturists, naturopaths, counselors, and others according to your own needs. Don't settle for good doctors. Find great doctors and terrific professionals. Find experts who click with you. Find people you trust.

● ● ● ● ● ● ● ● ● ● ● ● ● ● ● ● ●

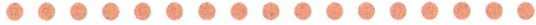

What to Look for in a GREAT Doctor

- Has training and experience in treating your specific type of back pain
- Is "board certified," so is fully credited in this specialty
- Has a good reputation in your community
- Listens well and responds well to you
- Encourages you to ask questions and gives you answers you understand
- Allows you to disagree and considers your ideas and opinions

PARTNER WITH YOUR DOCTORS

We've found that our wonderful docs appreciate that we take charge of our own pain. We acknowledge our responsibility for improving our health, but we require their expertise to pinpoint the cause of the pain and suggest solutions.

What's Causing the Pain?

Your job is to find out what's actually causing your pain, *if you can*. Keep seeing doctors and specialists, keep running tests, and keep digging until you find out what's essentially wrong with your back. You have great doctors and other professionals who are helping you, and you must keep trying to find what works for you. This is hard work that can be time-consuming and may be expensive, but it's worth it if you can pinpoint the problem or problems.

Most back pain is not just a single problem. It's often multiple problems that are happening in the same area at the same time. Sometimes, back pain doesn't originate in the back itself. "Referred Pain" means pain that starts in one place and is felt in

● ● ● ● ● ● ● ● ● ● ● ● ● ● ● ● ● ●

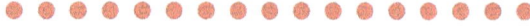

another. Hip pain, kidney pain, even heart attacks can present as back pain. You may find that your pain is not just from your back, but from somewhere else.

We want you to know that some people never get a firm diagnosis. This is a frustrating reality. But even not knowing exactly what's wrong, these people can learn to manage their symptoms and get on with their lives.

What Solutions Might Help?

Your doc should ask you something like: "What do you want?" The easy answer is something like "I want less pain," right? Right. But that's too vague. Specific goals will help your professionals to prescribe solutions. For instance:

- I want to walk in the park and play with my dog for an hour.
- I want to sit on the floor with my grandkids and get up without injuring myself.
- I want to get back to running a 5K with my friends.

We don't expect our docs to wave a magic wand and "fix" us. We let them know we're ready to do our part to help our own bodies. That means exercising, learning new ways to move, wearing a brace or taking off the brace, keeping therapy appointments, and doing what they suggest. This could include alternatives to surgery. You may find non-surgical treatments that work well for you.

For most of us, there is no single silver bullet that heals everything. A better strategy is to "nibble" at your pain.

● ● ● ● ● ● ● ● ● ● ● ● ● ● ● ● ●

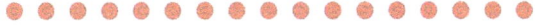

Tell Your Docs about Other Treatments You've Tried

During your first and subsequent visits to your doctor and surgeon, be sure to provide a summary of any alternative modalities you've tried (these are described in the next chapter). It will be helpful to write down the following, so your doc will know all the ways you're working to help your pain.

- What medications you've taken and how they affected your pain
- What treatments you've tried
- With what practice or organization
- How often and for how long
- What results you felt: any relief? 50% maybe? You felt better at first, but then it wasn't effective anymore?

We both use medical therapies beyond the scope of conventional medicine, and they're helpful additions to our doctors' plans. This mixing of therapies is called complementary or integrative or functional medicine.

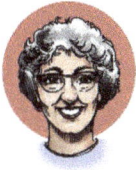

I regularly have sessions of dry needling and massage. I do Pilates, and I take supplements including turmeric for inflammation and magnesium for muscle spasms.

finding answers to your pain

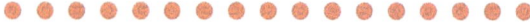

• • • • • • • • • • • • • • • • • •

> I go to a chiropractor regularly. I meditate and
> pray to release tension. I work with my
> naturopath to tailor supplements to my
> current needs. I also take magnesium, as
> well as calcium and glucosamine-chondroitin-
> MSM to protect my bones and joints from
> the steroid injections I get fairly often.

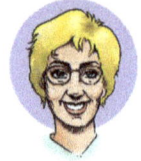

How to Describe Your Pain

How do you put into words what your pain feels like? How can you possibly explain to someone who isn't feeling it? We all need words and pictures that we can use; we need a common language with our medical professionals.

You may have seen the pain scale at the doctor's office:

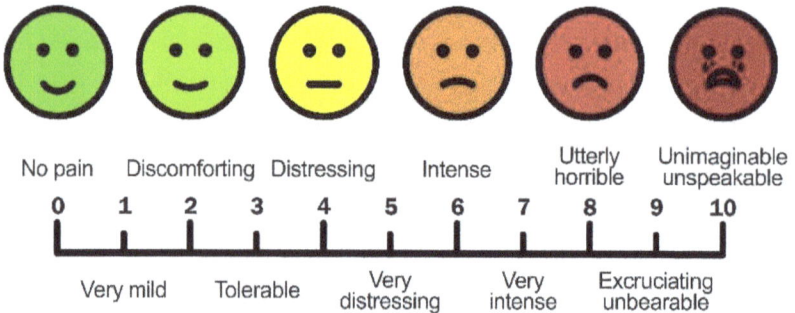

No pain	Discomforting	Distressing		Intense		Utterly horrible	Unimaginable unspeakable
0	1	2	3	4	5	6	7	8	9	10

Very mild   Tolerable   Very distressing   Very intense   Excruciating unbearable

We like this particular pain scale, because a 6 is "intense" and an 8 is "utterly horrible." It helps to have words associated with the numbers. But when you're in unrelenting, excruciating, life-changing pain, it may feel like you're off this chart. All of us need to be able to explain our pain more specifically than "it hurts." At the same time, remember that your doctors are used to hearing people exaggerate or even lie about their situation.

6

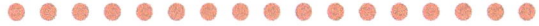

Here's part of a story from Firefighters and Paramedics
(FireFighterParamedicStories.Blogspot.com):

> I asked my patient to rate her pain on a scale of 1-10 if a 10
> was the most pain she had ever been in. This is a funny thing
> that goes on in the medical profession. We always ask the
> patient to rate the pain. **I generally don't care what they
> say their pain level is, their body language always tells me
> what I need to know.** So why do we ask? I digress.
> My patient said it was "a 10"! So I asked her if this was the
> single most painful event of her life. She looked at me as if
> I were stupid and said "No." So I tried to explain further.
> 'Think of the most pain you have ever been in, that is a 10.
> How is this pain compared to that?" "It's a 10," she said, still
> with that look of 'you're an idiot' plastered on her face.
> Really not the best tactic if you're trying to get some pain
> meds. At this point I gave up. She obviously isn't in much
> pain, if any at all.

So, instead of relying on a vague 10-point scale, we've learned
to have conversations with our docs instead. For instance, we
might say "On my 0-10 scale, I think a '10' would render me
unconscious. At a '9' you should call an ambulance, Given that
scale, today I'm a 5." This gets their attention.

If you say to your doctor "My pain is a 12!!!" and you were able
to get out of bed, dress, drive yourself to the doctor, sit upright
on the exam table, and chat … your pain isn't even a 9. Try not
to exaggerate and let them know you're trying not to
exaggerate. At the same time, make your needs known.

● ● ● ● ● ● ● ● ● ● ● ● ● ● ● ● ● ●

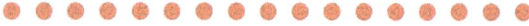

When my pain first started (remember I was 19), I wouldn't say "ouch" if a doctor hurt me during our appointment. Somehow, it seemed rude. I gritted my teeth (sometimes held my breath) and stayed quiet. A doctor who dug his thumbs into my broken vertebrae changed my mind. OUCH! Sometimes the doctor is more focused on what he's doing than on your reaction to it. You must say "THIS HURTS!" Otherwise, how will anyone know? This is true for massage therapists, chiropractors, and other professionals who will work on your back.

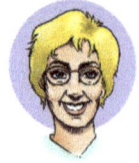

Help Lighten the Mood in the Waiting Room

Sitting in the doctor's waiting room can be agony, especially in those uncomfortable chairs. We're hoping for an answer to our problems, as are all the people around us. It's a very nerve-wracking time!

At the same time, doctors have a difficult job balancing the needs of all their patients. They try not to run late and make people wait. They also want to be sure to answer every patient's questions and address all concerns.

- Don't take out your frustration on the people who work there. Whatever is wrong, it's probably not the fault of the receptionist or the nurse or the PA or even the doctor.

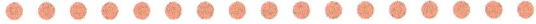

- Make your waiting time count. Try meditating or people-watching or listening to humorous videos (with your earbuds in). You may even want to bring your favorite book or tablet.

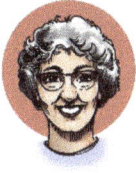

We never meet strangers! Both of us
find it easy to talk with people,
to joke a little, to share a story.
we try to lighten up the mood in
our doctors' waiting rooms.

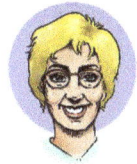

Keep Your Sense of Humor

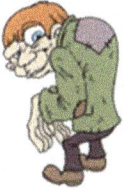

The hunchback didn't believe
he needed back surgery.
He now stands corrected.

For your back pain and for your life,
please try to keep your sense of humor.
Laughter relieves tension even better than crying.

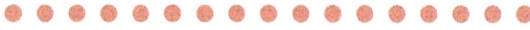

life with back pain

KEEP MOVING

A generation ago, back pain was treated with extended bed rest. Not anymore. Prolonged rest can actually increase pain. Here's what happens:

- Joints get less lubrication.
- Muscles weaken (you can see the difference after just two weeks of bed rest).
- Connective tissue stiffens.
- Discs in your back don't cushion as well.
- Toxins build up in your body.
- You get depressed or anxious, and …
- The pain gets worse.

Inactivity not only delays healing but also increases the risk of injury.

Instead, with your doctor's approval, get yourself up and moving, even just a little bit. Don't let fear rule you; the spine is truly one of the strongest parts of the human body. Your spine is comprised of solid bony blocks joined by discs to give them strength and flexibility. Those vertebrae are reinforced with

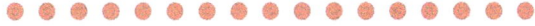

strong ligaments and surrounded by large powerful muscles to protect them. Your whole body is designed to move, including your spine. Don't stop living, just make adjustments for how you move.

WHEN BACK PAIN NEEDS IMMEDIATE ATTENTION

In America, 80% of us will have back pain at some point in our lives. Fortunately most back pain is not due to any serious disease. Many problems resolve themselves within a few days or weeks. Most cases resolve without surgery. However, sudden, new back pain may need immediate care. Here are some warning signs:

- You have a fever, chills, or other signs of infection.
- You lose control of bladder or bowel.
- Your leg (or both legs) suddenly won't move at all.
- The pain is severe enough to wake you up at night, and it's getting worse every minute that passes.

In these cases, please call 911 or see a doctor immediately.

AIDS FOR LIVING WITH BACK PAIN

Whether you're working to find your diagnosis or you already know what's wrong, your back hurts. That means your energy and stamina are lower right now. Please consider the following suggestions, which can make your life easier.

● ● ● ● ● ● ● ● ● ● ● ● ● ● ● ● ● ●

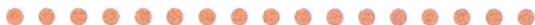

Apply for Handicapped Parking

You probably qualify for a Handicapped Parking Placard if:

- You're unable to walk without assistance, or
- You have mobility impairments such as arthritis, or neurological or orthopedic conditions.

Get and fill out an application for a "Disability License Placard" from your DMV and have it signed by your physician. Then take that filled-out form (or mail it) to your local DMV to obtain your placard. It can take a few weeks to process.

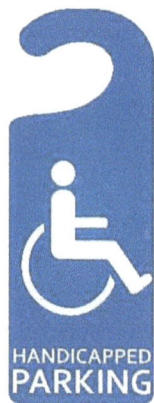

When your back hurts, your energy and your stamina are lower. Please use aids available to you so you can spend your energy on more important activities.

Use a Motorized Cart at Stores

Just like the handicapped parking space, please use the motorized cart at the grocery and other stores.

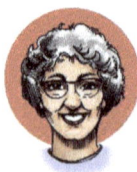

> The first time I got in a motorized cart, I drove straight into a display, knocking the whole thing over! I recommend that you learn how they work before you start shopping. ☺

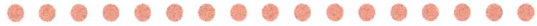

Consider Using a Walker

A walker can be very helpful when you need to walk for longer distances, or you're not sure of the terrain. If you have surgery, it will be useful in helping you feel secure as you're healing. There are many varieties of walkers available; please consult with your doctor or PT. Be sure to have it sized correctly for you. You don't want to hunch over to use your walker.

Try a TENS Unit

A TENS unit is a small, battery-powered box with electrode patches. You attach each patch where it hurts, and it produces a low voltage current. The electrical impulses stimulate nerve cells that block pain signals and reduce your perception of pain. It feels a little tingly, and you control the strength of the feeling.

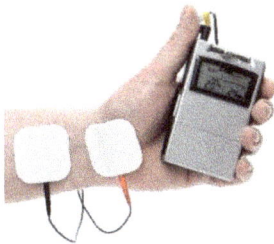

We've found that TENS can be a pleasant distraction and is good for short-term relief. It only helps while it's attached to your body and turned on.

Lighten Your Load

Be aware of the weight of things you're lifting, toting, arranging, or taking. We often don't consider the "everyday" carrying. Here's an example:

Grocery shopping can be exhausting. Walking through the store, standing in line to check out, and you're not finished when you get home! When you carry grocery bags into the house, plan ahead.

● ● ● ● ● ● ● ● ● ● ● ● ● ● ● ● ●

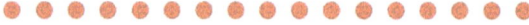

- You don't have to bring in everything all at once. If you're hurting, bring in the cold items and then take a break. The rest can wait.
- Be sure you aren't carrying too heavy a load on each trip. It's better to make more trips with fewer bags each time.

If you carry a purse or a wallet, try making it lighter and easier to carry. Women who carry a heavy bag on one shoulder will tend to lean over to compensate.

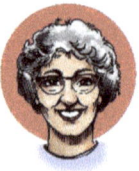

> I carry a smaller purse, although I cram it full of stuff. But it's not as heavy as the bag I used to carry!

> I weighed my purse and then took out five pounds of stuff until it now weighs just about two pounds. I don't even carry coins anymore... they're too heavy!

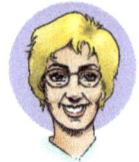

For men, please consider not carrying your wallet in your back pocket. The placement of back pockets can run along the sciatic nerves, and your wallet may be adding to your pain. Carry less with you or carry your wallet elsewhere.

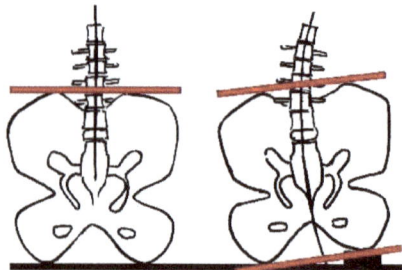

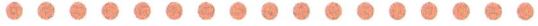

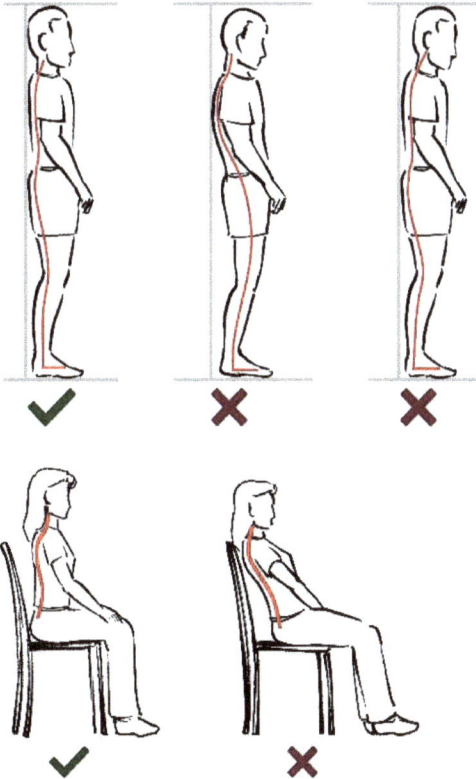

Improve Your Posture

Proper standing posture should look this way from the side: your ears over your shoulders, over hips, over knees, over ankles. You can test this by standing with your back against a wall. Your body should touch the wall at your butt, shoulder blades, and back of head. Everything else should have space between you and the wall.

While you're working on your posture, notice how you sit in a chair. No slouching!

Check Your Vision

If you wear glasses, especially if you wear bifocals, your head will tend to follow where your eyes look. If you must look up or down to see correctly, please visit your eye doctor. Your head needs to be correctly aligned, or your back may compensate and cause more pain.

● ● ● ● ● ● ● ● ● ● ● ● ● ● ● ● ●

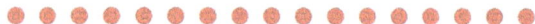

> When I went for my regular eye exam, the tech asked, "Why are you tilting your head back?" I said, "I didn't know I was tilting my head back!" Apparently, looking through the bifocal part of my glasses was giving me clearer vision and straining my neck at the same time. With new glasses, my neck feels much better!

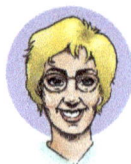

AIDS TO MANAGE YOUR PAIN AT HOME

Let Your Bed Be a Comfortable and Cozy Place

For many people, lying down in bed is the most comfortable position, and it feels great to "be flat." Don't fuss with too many pillows or too few. Make your bed what you need for yourself right now.

Have a Supportive, Comfortable Mattress

Only you can tell what's right for you. Mattresses have come a long way in the last few years. If you haven't tried out new mattresses, then this is a great time to upgrade.

Find a Pillow You Love

Pillows are truly an individual preference. Remember, getting proper rest will be a part of your healing journey. You should sleep on your back or side, not on your belly.

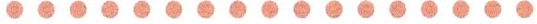

Lie on Your Side with a Pillow Between Your Knees

The knee pillow will help you be more comfortable and will keep your hips in a good relative position. See the illustration:

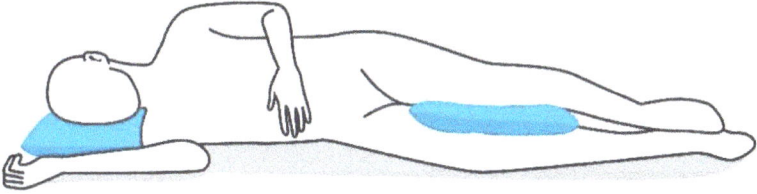

Lie on Your Back with a Pillow Under Your Knees

This position provides a "pelvic tilt," where your lower back is a little rounded. This should feel good, and this position helps create relaxation. See the illustration:

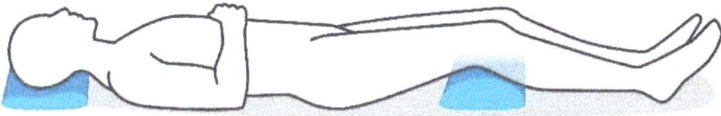

Of course, as you're sleeping, pillows and blankets may go every which way, but don't worry. Just sleep as comfortably as you can each night. Good sleep is essential for good health.

● ● ● ● ● ● ● ● ● ● ● ● ● ● ● ● ● ●

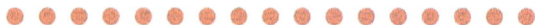

> For the pillow under my head, I slice up a memory foam pillow to make the perfect shape for me, whether sleeping on back or side. When I lie on my side, I like a pillow between my knees, and another pillow to hug. This way, my upper arm doesn't have to stretch all the way down to the mattress. Plus, I find it emotionally comforting...

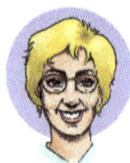

Get a High Toilet Seat or Seat Extender

There are many variations of higher toilet seats available; you choose what works best for you. Some come with "arms," which can also be helpful when your legs feel weak. Some are temporary and some are permanent.

Put Grab Bars in Your Shower and Toilet Area

These are safety features we think every home should have. They'll give you confidence in a slippery area, and you can hold on while you shower. They can be permanently mounted to the wall studs or temporarily attached with suction cups. Those with a lockable latch are stronger, and they come in various lengths. Be sure not to mount a suction bar on a grout line, because it won't stick securely. You may even want to install grab bars down your hallways – consider any place where you may need some extra help.

Have a Non-Slip Mat in Your Bath/Shower Area

We think every home should have this safety aid.

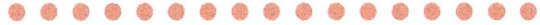

Use a Long-Handled Bath Brush

This will help you reach your backside and below your knees while you're in the shower.

Buy a Grabber/Reacher

This will help you reach down or up in any room for many purposes. We like the kind with a "locking grip" so your hand strength isn't taxed while holding onto that can of soup or whatever you're grabbing. Try one with silicone or rubber on the insides of the "pincher," so your item doesn't slip out.

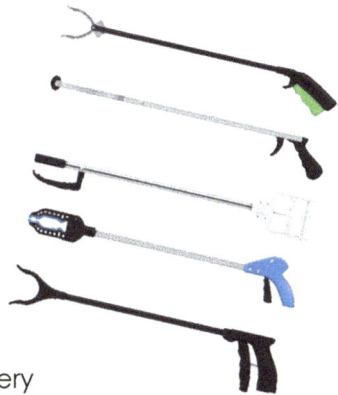

Have at least one long one and one short. Lori has a "grabber" in every room! They're not as strong as we'd like, but they're still very helpful.

Try Temporary Relief with Lidocaine or CBD or Pain Patches, Gels, Creams, Sprays, and Roll-ons

There are many kinds of pain relief to apply to your skin. Although we don't expect these to completely relieve your pain, they can help some. Try several and see what works for you. Temporary relief is still relief.

Soak in Hot Water

Fill your bathtub with 1 cup of Epsom salts, 1 cup baking soda, and 1/4 cup powdered ginger. The magnesium in Epsom salts will relax muscles, the baking soda and ginger will help remove inflammatory toxins. Stay in the water until you're sweating.

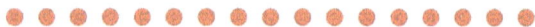

If you use Epsom salts, you'll want to rinse off the salty water. And, of course, please be careful getting in and out of the tub.

Alternate Hot and Cold
Cold is good for swelling and inflammation, especially if you've overworked or fallen. Heat is good for muscles in spasm or for getting circulation into an area. The application of heat for 15 minutes, followed by cold for 15 minutes, can be surprisingly effective to relieve pain. You can repeat this as needed.
Try ice packs, frozen peas, heating pads, or packs that are used for both hot and cold. Even a sock filled with rice or beans can be put in the microwave and provides lasting warm heat.

Stop Smoking
If you're still smoking, we encourage you to quit. As ex-smokers ourselves, we sympathize. But smoking does damage to more than just your lungs. We were surprised to learn that smoking has a very negative effect not just on our lungs, but on our whole bodies. Some surgeons won't operate on smokers. It decreases oxygen delivery to healing tissues and creates unnecessary risk.

PREVENT FALLING
During a time when one part of the body is in distress, the rest of the body works harder to compensate. This is the time to be extra vigilant with your whole body. Falls happen suddenly, often when you aren't paying attention. **Stop and think before you move.** Here are some tips:

- Walk carefully. Look where you're going. Pick up your feet, don't shuffle. Watch for uneven pavement, especially curbs. Try not to do other things while you're

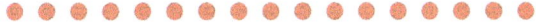

walking. For instance, don't walk and read your phone at the same time.

- Stand up slowly, allowing your hips to hinge and then straighten. Once you're standing, pause a moment to regain your balance. This will help prevent dizziness.

- Wear properly fitting shoes with non-skid soles. Loose shoes or worn-out soles increase your risk of falling.

- Remove area rugs to avoid tripping.

- Add lighting in your home if there are dark hallways or areas where you regularly walk, especially at steps or changes from carpet to smooth flooring.

- Keep electrical cords out of the way.

- Improve your balance. Tai Chi, or Ai Chi in the water, is famous for helping balance. Video courses from Silver Sneakers are also targeted for better balance.

- Improve your leg strength. Some simple exercises can strengthen your ankles, your knees, your hips, and will help keep you from falling. Ask your physical therapist or doctor.

To improve my balance, I began a new habit. While I brush my teeth, I stand on one foot. I've progressed from just lifting one heel, to actually taking my whole foot off the floor. I'm improving!

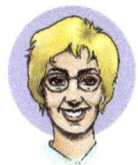

● ● ● ● ● ● ● ● ● ● ● ● ● ● ● ● ● ●

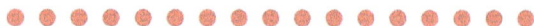

SOME SURPRISING SIDE EFFECTS OF LIVING WITH PAIN

It's a strange phenomenon, but we've discovered some positive changes to our lives. These transformations have happened because of (or sometimes in spite of) the pain we've endured.

Gratitude

We've experienced days when we were unable to get out of bed. When having a shower and putting on clothes was a big goal for the day, and worthy of celebration if we managed it. On days when the pain was overwhelming, without an end in sight, it was easy to succumb to sadness and apathy.

When we began to feel better, we became incredibly grateful for the ability to get out of bed on most days. Now we're happy to live just a "normal" life. For someone who is NOT in pain, how happy are they to see "normal"? Those of us in pain are thrilled just to go out to lunch with friends. We're more grateful for "normal" than ever before.

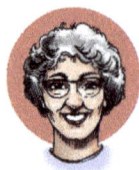

> I believe happiness is a decision I make. No matter what kind of day I'm having, it's never as bad as I think it is. Change my trajectory, and something unpleasant has turned into gratitude. Take the good with the bad and find joy in the little things.

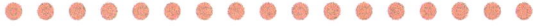

Re-prioritizing

When life is "normal," our priorities are all over the place.
We live for work, play, home, entertainment, relationships,
exercise, fun, growth, and new experiences, pushing our
boundaries of comfort. When pain enters our lives, our priorities
become quite simple. Our first priority, whether we like it or not,
is our own bodies. We must focus on ourselves, resting,
stretching, gently moving, in the hopes that our lives can then
include some other things. Learning self-care is a positive
addition to our perspective.

Compassion

Now that we've lived in pain, we can truly see other people in
pain. We're grateful to be able to greet a stranger who's using
a cane, or open a door for someone with a walker, or just give
a smile to someone who's limping. We're reminded of our own
days when just walking in the door was a big accomplishment.

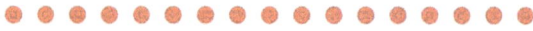

alternatives to surgery

THERAPIES

Since back pain is often caused by multiple problems, it's very seldom that one pain reliever (pills, or surgery, or exercises, or injections) will completely fix what hurts. As mentioned, a better strategy is to "nibble" at your pain. Find something that helps part of your pain and add that to your life. Then find another thing and add that. Pretty soon, your pain will be smaller. As you continue to find things that relieve some of your pain, eventually you'll come to a place where you can live well with these remedies. This is our hope for you.

Each unique body responds differently to pain, so please try some different solutions, and see how your body reacts. Here are some therapies that have helped us, along with information to do further research for yourself.

Physical Therapy

Your doctor can refer you to a physical therapist (PT), and you want an outstanding one. Some will work with you in the gym doing supervised exercises. Some PTs will manipulate your back with their hands to stretch and align. Some use "dry needling,"

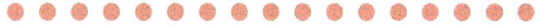

a process of inserting tiny needles deep into muscles that cannot be reached in any other way. It may be uncomfortable for a moment. There's usually a "zing" and a twitch just before the muscle relaxes. Physical or occupational therapists (OTs) teach you how to move your body and give you exercises according to your specific needs. Visit *APTA.org* or *AOTA.org*.

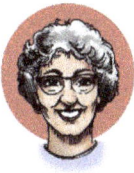

We really bonded as friends and "sisters" when we discovered that we each see the same wonderful physiotherapist. **Her philosophy is to help us become well enough to not need her.** We go back to her occasionally for "tune ups"!

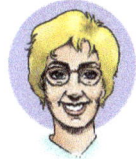

Gentle Exercise

This can include stretching, walking, even gentle yoga. We both do some simple exercises at home, and they help us feel better. When we neglect exercise, our bodies let us know. Your PT can recommend what exercises are right for you, how many repetitions to do, and how often to work out. Once you learn your exercises, incorporate them into your life. Do them regularly. Really. Regularly.

If you try an exercise class or follow a class on your TV or computer, don't try to keep up with the teacher. Be very aware of your own body and its needs and limitations right now. We recommend that you aim for about half of what the class is doing — move half as fast, do half as many, reach half as far. Better to start out very slowly than to overdo on the first day and pay for it later.

● ● ● ● ● ● ● ● ● ● ● ● ● ● ● ● ●

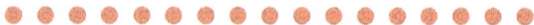

Water Exercise

Water relieves the force of gravity that's constantly pressing on our spines, so we feel relief just by being in a pool. The buoyancy of the water helps us feel lighter and allows us to move easily in ways we can't on land. It's good for our backs and our whole bodies. Find a gentle water exercise class, or just get in the pool and walk and play around by yourself. Let your body tell you what feels good and what doesn't for today.

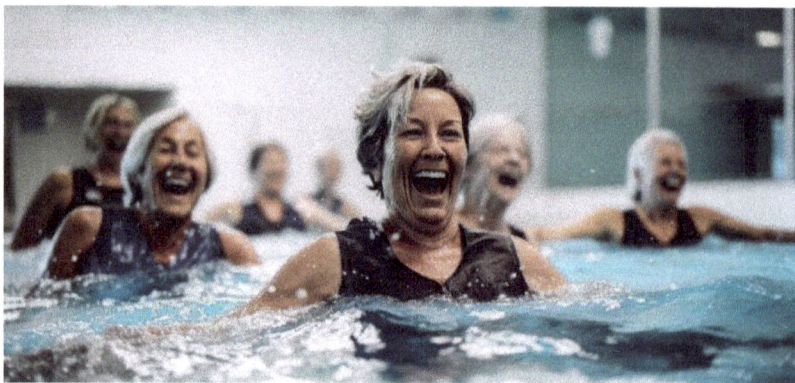

In 2010, I tried a water exercise class that was offered at my local YMCA. That experience began a routine that's been regular for me ever since. Every time I leave the pool, I feel better than when I entered the water. Now I teach that class (plus two others), and it's helping not just me but many other people who are living with pain.

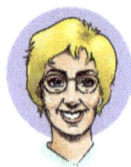

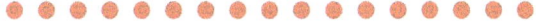

Chiropractic

Chiropractors specialize in the health of your spine. They'll adjust your back with their hands and/or devices in order to correct imbalances in your spine. Many chiropractors also use lasers, electrical stimulation, or other methods to relieve pain. Visit *ACAToday.org*.

Acupuncture

Get a recommendation from a medical professional for an excellent practitioner of acupuncture. Acupuncturists treat a wide variety of ills, including pain, using very thin needles. The treatment really doesn't hurt! In fact, it's often relaxing. Visit *MedicalAcupuncture.org*, or *AAAOMOnline.org, or NCCAOM.org* to find an acupuncturist who's certified and has a good reputation among medical professionals.

Therapeutic Massage

We enjoy many kinds of massage, but a therapeutic massage can really help our pain. The therapist can manipulate joints, muscles, and connective tissue (fascia) to promote better blood flow, alignment, and pain relief.

Pain Medication

Conscientious use of prescription painkillers can be positively life-changing. A good pain management practitioner can give you options, including opioid and non-opioid pain relievers, and they can answer your questions. Most people don't want to take pain medications, but please don't rule them out. Keep an open mind as you're investigating your options.

● ● ● ● ● ● ● ● ● ● ● ● ● ● ● ● ●

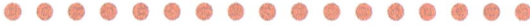

Injections and Ablations

In addition to medications given by mouth, pain management doctors can also offer targeted injections and ablations.

Injections place a small amount of medicine (usually a steroid) in a specific place to relieve pain. The relief can last from a few days to a few years. During a nerve ablation, officially known as Endoscopic Rhizotomy, the

EPIDURAL STEROID INJECTION

nerve is deadened. Typically, an ablation is used in hopes of a longer period of relief.

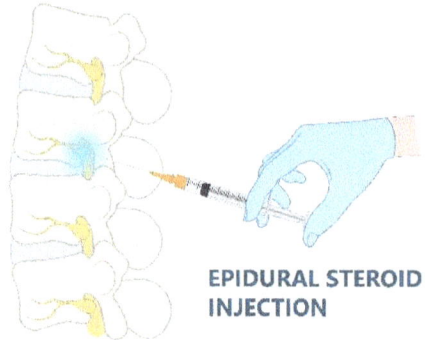

Spinal Cord Stimulator

A spinal cord stimulator is an implanted device that treats chronic severe pain, and it's usually an option when other means of controlling pain are unsuccessful. First, you'll have a trial period when your doc hopes to achieve 50% reduction in pain.

If you continue, you'll undergo a small surgical procedure. Under your skin, doc will implant electrodes that send low levels of electricity into your spinal cord. These electrodes are connected to a battery implanted in your hip. The stimulator is programmed by your medical team with a separate controller. Spinal stimulators don't heal your source of pain; they change how your brain interprets it.

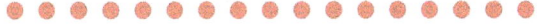

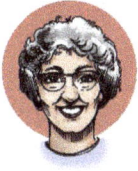

> My implanted stimulator gave me great pain relief for a couple of years. Then I took a hard fall, and the wires inside stopped working as well. We tried several program changes, but the stimulator just didn't work anymore. Since then, it's just been turned off. Even though it doesn't help me anymore, and it can't be removed, I would still recommend trying a spinal cord stimulator.

Counseling

Living with pain is an emotional rollercoaster. A good counselor can help us have hope and can change the negative "inner dialogue" that makes things worse. We've found that a positive attitude helps bring about pain relief, while stress and anxiety can increase our pain. Pain Psychologists are specially trained to help those of us who live with pain. Visit *AAPainPsychology.org*.

Meditation

Bodies in pain experience "fight or flight" response, tensing our muscles and preparing for action. Chronic pain leaves us all constantly "on edge," with increased production of cortisol and adrenaline. Meditation can help calm both our minds and our bodies. For some people, the quiet and calm of daily meditation is sufficient to relieve much of their pain. At the least, it can be a few moments of peace and rest.

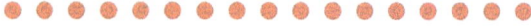

Meditation was difficult for me at first; it was hard to slow down my thoughts. But I listened to recordings from Jon Kabat-Zinn called "meditation for pain relief," and I've found it really helps calm down my mind and my body. Like most worthwhile activities, practice improves performance.

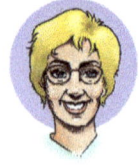

Vitamins and Supplements

Supplements and over-the-counter medicines can help relieve pain. For instance, turmeric is a well-known anti-inflammatory. Before you take vitamins or supplements, please see a knowledgeable source like a naturopath or holistic healer who is well-versed in supplementation. Naturopaths don't specialize in pain relief, but they're concerned with the health of your entire body. They often have gentler, non-prescription treatments. Please confirm with your docs and pharmacist that the supplements will not interfere with your prescription meds. Your pharmacist can be a real ally in this area. Visit *Naturopathic.org*.

New Therapies as Time Progresses

The medical community is very invested in creating and trying new therapies, especially for back pain. Please continue to ask and search for new ways to relieve pain. We're hopeful for the future of back pain treatment.

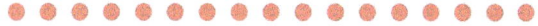

DIFFERENT TYPES OF DOCTORS
PROVIDE DIFFERENT PERSPECTIVES

As you're seeking alternatives to surgery, you may want to visit different kinds of doctors, since each will have its own area of specialization.

Orthopedic Specialists & Surgeons

Orthopedic docs treat your bones, muscles, and joints. Many specialize in certain areas — the knee doc, the shoulder doc, etc. They also work on backs. Visit *AAOMed.org* and *AAOS.org*.

Neurologists and Neurosurgeons

These are physicians who specialize in the diagnosis and treatment of disorders of the central and peripheral nervous system — the brain and spine. Neurologists specialize in head and back pain. They work on nerves, which convey pain messages. Visit *MYANA.org* and *AANS.org*.

Osteopathic Doctors

Doctors of Osteopathy, or DOs, are MDs who believe there's more to good health than the absence of pain or disease. Their whole-person approach to medicine focuses on prevention, helping promote the body's natural tendency toward health and self-healing. Visit *Osteopathic.org*.

Rheumatologists

Rheumatologists treat arthritis and other diseases that cause pain, swelling, and stiffness in your body. They can diagnose and treat auto-immune issues. Visit *Rheumatology.org*.

alternatives to surgery

● ● ● ● ● ● ● ● ● ● ● ● ● ● ● ● ● ●

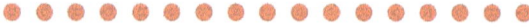

Sports Medicine Physicians

Sports medicine docs work with a variety of patients, from youth athletes and weekend warriors to elite athletes and regular folks, too. They have significant specialized training in both the treatment and prevention of illness and injury to help you achieve your personal best and lead a healthier lifestyle. Visit *AMSSM.org*.

Pain Management Doctors

Pain medicine specialists treat many kinds of pain, including pain that doesn't have a clear diagnosis. They can recommend physical therapy, oral medications, injections, and many other resources for reducing or eliminating pain. Physiatrists or rehabilitation physicians are MDs who treat pain related to nerves, muscles, and joints. They are often anesthesiologists or other MDs who have pursued additional training in pain management. Visit *PainMed.org, ASIPP.org, and USPainFoundation.org*.

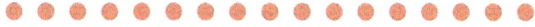

what's next?

NOW WHAT?

Now you have good information about your back and how it's responded to some alternatives. It's time to discuss with your doctor and your family and make your decision about surgery. Weigh the pros and cons.

For some of you, the decision to have surgery will be simplified.

- Some conditions, like broken bones, require surgery — you can't live your fullest life without it.

- Some of you will find that your pain can't be fixed with surgery. There's no need to consider surgery since it won't help.

- Some of you will have found enough relief from the pain that you're content to live without surgery. You may be comfortable not having surgery at this time and visiting the doc again in six months.

If you can't do most of your activities most of the time, and nothing has relieved your pain enough, it may be time to consider surgery.

● ● ● ● ● ● ● ● ● ● ● ● ● ● ● ● ● ● ●

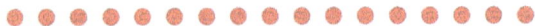

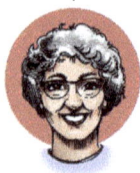

> My doctor asked me, "When did you finally know
> you needed spine surgery?" My answer was,
> "When my pain negatively affected my life,
> and nothing else had worked." I had tried
> other treatments, and I had great
> confidence in my surgeon.

> When my back pain first started, I spent a year
> trying non-surgical techniques, and nothing
> worked. My medical tests showed definitively
> broken vertebrae. For me, spinal fusion was
> absolutely necessary.

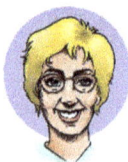

Before you agree to surgery, we recommend getting a second opinion from another surgeon in a different practice.

It's beneficial to have another doctor examine you and review your test results. Either you'll get another medical option to try, or you'll get confirmation that the original recommendation is the best course of action for you.

In addition, ask your friends and family for their input. We're certain that you know someone who knows someone who knows a great back doctor. You'll hear some interesting stories, and you may be encouraged about your own situation.

● ● ● ● ● ● ● ● ● ● ● ● ● ● ● ● ● ●

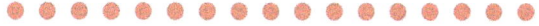

If you decide to have surgery, please keep reading.
Preparation for and expectations about your surgery are key
to your best results. We've been through surgeries, and we can
help you anticipate and make arrangements to allow for easier
and faster healing.

If you decide NOT to have surgery, please keep reading.
You can read and consider the suggestions around surgery,
and then all the rest of the book will help you live better with
your imperfect back.

your surgeon

YOUR BACK IS IN YOUR SURGEON'S HANDS

Now you've met with several doctors and other medical professionals. Together you've decided surgery is necessary. You really like your surgeon, and you feel confident putting your back *literally* into those hands.

Expectations

Managing our expectations as patients is incredibly important to recovery. If you're expecting to never have back pain again, then you'll be disappointed. You need to be hopeful but realistic, just as you expect your doctors to be.

Docs Are People Too

Let's also remember that our doctors are human beings, they are not God. They work hard to figure out what's wrong with our backs, and what we need to feel better. Let's lend them some kindness and not expect them to work miracles.

Did you know that the average spine surgeon sees 30 patients a day in the office? Also, for surgeons, only about 30% of their patients require surgery. The rest are treated with other methods. The docs don't have as much time as they'd like to spend with you as their patient, but they're doing the best they can.

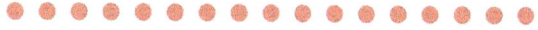

One of our docs shared this with us:

> *I had a hard time keeping up with charting each visit in real time, since I wanted to give my complete attention to my patient. So, I entered information into the electronic record during evenings or weekends. This was hard on me as well as on my family.*

Since our doctors are imperfect but doing their best, it's incumbent upon us to find out how we can best help ourselves.

SURGEONS' ADVICE TO ALL OF US

We asked our favorite surgeons how we could help them, and what exactly was our responsibility as patients. Here's what they told us.

Help Your Doctor Help You

Our doctors said they need us to **fully participate in the process**. Surgeons have no magic wand. Doctors can solve anatomical problems, but your contribution to your own care is most important. Whatever choices you have, whether surgical, conservative, or whatever... **as patients we all must do the work.** We can't sit idly by and expect the docs to "fix us." It doesn't work that way.

Medical care is a partnership between the patient, the surgeon, and the medical team. It's important that you understand what to expect, but also what is expected of you as the patient. Self-care is extremely important. This includes good nutrition, getting plenty of exercise, not smoking, and taking medications as prescribed.

Operations are performed to solve a specific surgical problem. It's always great when results are better than expected,

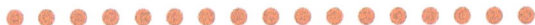

and it's disappointing when the opposite happens. Doctors do their best for us. As patients, we must do our part to make our surgery a success!

Take Charge Yourself

Our docs said our responsibility as patients includes many things. First, self-education. The better educated you are about your health conditions and options, including how your body works, the better choices you can make. The ability to communicate your needs and concerns is also extremely important, as is asking questions. Speak up and keep asking until you understand the explanation. Take charge of your own health, as we advised earlier. Having support from family and friends helps with that.

THINKING ABOUT YOUR SURGERY

How much do you want to know? If you want to know every detail, ask your doctor to provide all the particulars. If you *don't* want to know, tell your doc that.

> Before my surgery in 1984 (long before internet searching was available), I went to my local hospital and delved into their medical library. The research there was invaluable for me, and although I couldn't understand every word, I learned the basics about surgical options at that time. So, when my surgeon met me in my hospital room, I could ask him intelligent questions and get my answers in detail. Not knowing is scary for me!

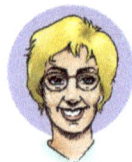

● ● ● ● ● ● ● ● ● ● ● ● ● ● ● ● ●

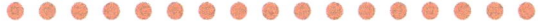

*We recommend that you bring someone with you
to all your medical appointments.*

It's always good to have a second pair of ears while you're with
the doc. If you can't have someone in person, use FaceTime,
Skype, Zoom, or whatever virtual program works for you.
Sometimes we ask if we can record our conversation to
review at home later.

QUESTIONS ABOUT YOUR SURGERY

Before your appointment, write down questions for your
surgeon. Here are some that we have asked, in no
particular order:

- How long will I be in the hospital?
- What kind of pain should I expect after surgery? How will
  that pain be managed, both in hospital and at home?
- Is going to a rehabilitation facility a good idea for me?
  If so, how long and where will I be in rehab? Here are
  reasons why we like rehab time after surgery:
  - You'll have a safe place for your first few days.
    You'll have nothing on your "to do" list and people
    available to help you 24 hours a day.
  - You can learn tricks for living with your specific
    problems. Information from the PT and OT is
    invaluable for better and faster healing.
  - When you get home, your care will be easier.
    Since you've had a few days to get up and about,
    you're not as fragile as you were just after surgery.
- Will there be physical therapy once I get home?
- If I were your mother, would you recommend this
  same approach?

your surgeon

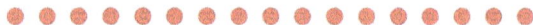

- How long until I can return to work or to my "normal" life?
- If you're a person who wants details:
  - What would you consider a positive outcome of my surgery? What would be a neutral outcome? A poor outcome?
  - How many of *these* surgeries have you done? What is your percentage of success? Can we agree on a definition of "success" in my case?

before
your
surgery

PREPARE

Now it's time to prepare for surgery. Planning will provide you peace of mind and make your recuperation easier. The goal is to make you as comfortable as possible so you can heal. Patients and caregivers who have a thorough understanding of what to expect from surgery will have less anxiety in the days and weeks surrounding it.

GET YOUR WORKPLACE READY

Plan enough time off work, even if you work from home. Your doctor should tell you approximately how much time you should take off work, based on your specific circumstances. This may be revised after your surgery. If you work from home, then allow yourself enough time to recuperate at home before you start actually working at home. You may be tempted to work, since you're still at home, but your body needs rest and measured activity. Please allow yourself that time.

Please actually take time off from work. Our bodies require time to rest, especially after surgery. You're going to need time to heal; if you don't give your body the time it needs, then you risk

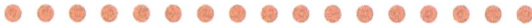

● ● ● ● ● ● ● ● ● ● ● ● ● ● ● ● ● ●

not healing properly. Even if your outcome is *ideal*, your body has still been through trauma and needs time.

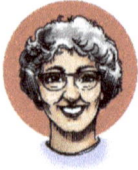

> We both tend to be overachievers. It's not easy for us to say "no" to a good project. One habit we both had to break was continuing to work even during severe pain. Sometimes you have no choice but to push through the pain and do the work. But, as best you can, try to stop and rest.

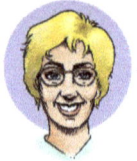

Avoid a mountain of work when you return. Is there a co-worker who can cover some of your work? Someone who could just answer your communications? Use automated answering for your email and voicemail if that's available to you. Don't try to do it all yourself.

GET YOUR HOME READY

Making some temporary changes to your home will make things easier for you as you recover. Here are some things we've done that were helpful. Your doctor may have other ideas to add. We've put a shopping list together at the end of this chapter.

Your Entire Home

Clear a safe walking path for yourself in every room. No rugs or changes of height, nothing on the floors — just clear, even space to get you from one place to another.

Think about the stairs. Do you have to go upstairs? If so, talk with your doctor. Perhaps arranging a room downstairs would be

●●●●●●●●●●●●●●●●●●

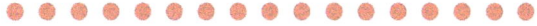

advisable for these first few days, when stairs will be difficult to navigate. Your doctor can issue a prescription to a medical supply store for you to rent a hospital bed for a week.

Your Bathroom

When you're fresh from your surgery, moving around may be painful or awkward. Here are some tools and techniques that can help you.

Consider renting a chair toilet. For the first few days, rather than having to walk from your bed to the bathroom, it may be more comfortable to have a chair toilet in your room.

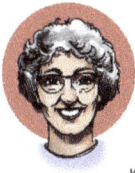

I rented a chair toilet so I wouldn't even have to walk the few steps to the bathroom. After a few days, I moved the rented toilet to over my regular toilet seat. It provided a taller seat and gave me arms to push on. That helped me stand up.

Get bottom wipers/toilet aids. It can be awkward to reach behind you to wipe your bottom, so try a bottom wiper. It's a long handle, designed to be used between your legs. Some are designed with pre-moistened wipes attached. Some will have you wrap toilet paper around the end first.

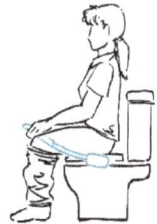

Consider a bidet. It's a sanitary device that's connected to your toilet and provides a stream of water to rinse before wiping. Many people feel cleaner when using a bidet. They now come in a wide range of prices and functions. The most affordable bidets don't heat the water before spraying (chilly ☺).

43

● ● ● ● ● ● ● ● ● ● ● ● ● ● ● ● ● ●

You may also try using a "peri-bottle," which is like an inexpensive portable bidet.

Rent or purchase a shower bench or shower seat. Sitting down while showering feels like a luxury, and it makes the whole process easier and safer. This will be helpful for the first few days, and you may find it beneficial for your life after surgery.

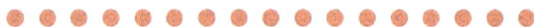

Your Kitchen

Place things you use often on your countertop. That way, you won't have to search or lean. Whatever you'll use most: things like coffee or tea, bread, a small pan for cooking. Choose what's right for you.

Use disposable plates, cutlery, and cups for a little while. No need to do dishes during recovery. Remember you're trying to make things as easy as possible on yourself.

Prepare meals or buy ready-to-eat meals in advance. You won't want to cook for a while after your surgery, so having prepared meals in the freezer will make eating easier for you. This is also a good idea for your friends who want to help but don't know what you need.

Your Bedroom

Place comfy clothing within easy reach. You'll want stretchy clothes that are easily taken on/off, and you don't want to fight with heavy drawers or hangers.

Consider renting a hospital bed. Especially if your bedroom is upstairs, you may want to make a temporary bedroom downstairs, and a hospital bed will make sleeping and moving around easier.

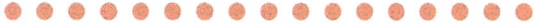

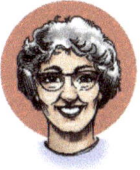

> I rented a hospital bed after my first surgery and found it so helpful that I did it again after my last surgery. Not only could I easily raise and lower my head, but raising and lowering the entire bed made it easier for me to get in and out. Holding onto the railings helped me turn over.

Try portable rails on your bed. If you don't rent a hospital bed, you may like portable bed rails for adults. This will give you the rails for safety and to hold onto while you turn over.

GET YOUR FAMILY READY

Arrange some caregiving for the first few days. At least have a family member or friend come check on you in person every day and call regularly. If you don't have a caregiver nearby, please consider hiring an aide for your first few days at home. This is another good reason to spend a few days in rehab, if that's an option for you.

Have a conversation with everyone who lives in your home. How are they feeling? Do they have questions? Are they scared? Are they ready to help when you get back home? It can be helpful for children to have some information before your surgery.

● ● ● ● ● ● ● ● ● ● ● ● ● ● ● ● ●

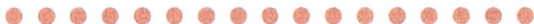

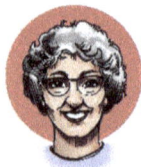

My daughter tacked post-it notes around
my home. The notes not only reminded me
to have good posture, but that I was
loved. Things like:

Stand Tall   No Slouching
Shoulders Back   Is your brace on?

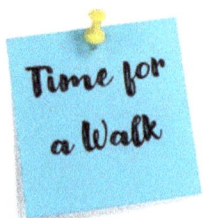

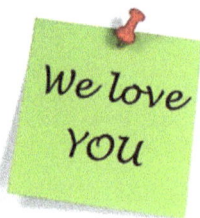

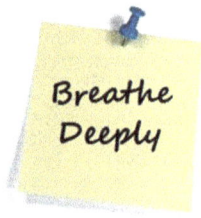

Time for
a Walk

We love
YOU

Breathe
Deeply

GET YOURSELF READY

How are you feeling about this process? Would it be helpful
to talk with someone? To sort through the changes in your life
because of your pain? Counseling or good friends will be very
valuable during this time.

Allow time to manage trauma. Back pain, with or without
surgery, is traumatic to your body and mind. Take some time
to feel your losses, your lessened activity, the heartache of now
having to "think about your body." Your life has changed,
and you're going to be OK.

Prepare yourself to be recovering for a little while. If it's your
nature to "get up and go," this may be difficult. Your body
will need time to heal and adjust.

● ● ● ● ● ● ● ● ● ● ● ● ● ● ● ● ● ● ●

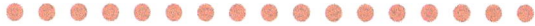

Remember everyone is different, and we each need different things. If you need time alone, ask for that. If you need a hug, ask for that.

Talk to people who have had the surgery you're about to have. Ask them questions. Here are some:

- How was your recovery?
- How did the pain after your surgery compare to the pain before your surgery?
- How long did it take to resume normal activities?
- How is your mobility now?
- What activities can you enjoy? What activities are still too much?
- If you had known what you know now, would you still have had the surgery?

Learn to ask for help. This can be surprisingly difficult. It's humbling to admit that we need help. Most of us are used to being independent, but life is made up of both giving and receiving help. Try not to be embarrassed to ask for what you actually need.

Allow friends or family to help. You may know people who want to help but don't know what to do. You can manage this easily with a list of tasks that could be handled by someone else. Your list may be different from ours:

- Cleaning Bathrooms
- Vacuuming or Sweeping
- Mowing Lawn
- Watering Plants

before your surgery

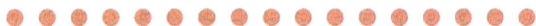

● ● ● ● ● ● ● ● ● ● ● ● ● ● ● ● ●

- Laundry
- Changing Sheets
- Pet Care
- Meal Delivery

Asking for help may feel uncomfortable. Do it anyway. Let your friends and family love you in these tangible ways.

Work with a physical therapist to improve the strength and flexibility of your back before your surgery. We hope you already have a great PT. Some are covered by insurance, some are not. Some are worth every penny you have to pay.

Strengthening your body before your surgery will help your body recover after surgery.

Your PT can provide exercises specific to your body's needs. The overall purpose of physical therapy is to increase your range of motion, your endurance, and to correct muscle imbalances. Strengthening posture and core muscles is vital. PT will help improve your daily life functions for home, for work, for play.

Consider banking your blood. Your doctor will know whether you may need a blood transfusion during your surgery. If so, you should consider having your own blood on hand. If you don't need it during your surgery, then it can be donated to a blood bank.

● ● ● ● ● ● ● ● ● ● ● ● ● ● ● ● ● ● ●

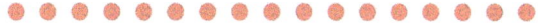

PACK FOR THE HOSPITAL

Most things are provided for you at the hospital, but it's nice to have some of your own things there.

Paperwork

- Driver's license
- Insurance card
- Medicine list
- Advance Directive / Living Will / Medical Power of Attorney
- Family and/or friends' phone numbers

Once you've checked in to the hospital, give these valuable documents to a friend or family member for safekeeping.

Comfort

- Socks or slip-on shoes, with slip-resistant soles
- Lip balm and lotion (it's very dry in the hospital)
- Loose-fitting stretchy clothes and undergarments
- Phone and phone charger
- Book or tablet or Kindle
- Pen/pencil and paper to write down questions or things you need to do. Record the medicines prescribed on discharge (frequency and dose) to reference when you get home.
- Look at your bedside table and bring things you use regularly.
- **Bring this book**. *It will encourage you while you're in the hospital, and you can remind yourself of the next steps in your recuperation.*

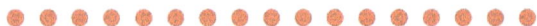

SHOPPING *List*

☐	Walker
☐	Chair Toilet or Toilet Seat Extender
☐	Bottom Wipers
☐	Bidet or Peri Bottle
☐	Grab Bars for Bathroom Areas
☐	Non-slip Mats
☐	Shower Bench or Chair
☐	Long-Handled Bath Brush
☐	Disposable Plates, Cups, Silverware
☐	Ready-to-Eat meals
☐	Reacher/Grabber
☐	Hospital Bed
☐	Portable Rails
☐	
☐	
☐	

Check with your insurance to see if they supply some of these items for you, especially the walker, hospital bed, or bed rails.

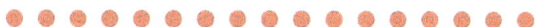

in
the
hospital

HEALING AFTER SURGERY

Some people wake up from surgery already sensing that their underlying pain is gone, and we hope this is the case for you. However, most people will have additional pain at first, and then a gradual reduction over the next few weeks and months.

The nurses and techs will get you out of bed quickly, probably before you feel ready. Do whatever they request of you. Right after surgery, you'll need to work through the pain as best you can. Listen to your body, and rest when you need it.

Pain Medicine

If you're in pain, ask for pain medicine. Don't be shy. It is much easier to prevent pain than to try to manage it once you're really hurting. So don't wait until the pain is severe before getting medicine. You'll also take less medicine overall because you're "staying ahead" of the pain. This will continue to be true during your first few days at home.

At the same time, don't take medicine just because "it's time." If you don't have pain when it's time for your next dose, then don't take those meds right away. Listen to your body, and let it

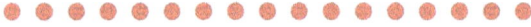

dictate what you need. Ultimately, you'll learn how much medicine you need and at what times. But for now, let the nurses and techs take care of you.

Write down the times you take pain meds while you're in the hospital. You can use this as a guide when you get home.

Try to sleep as much as you can. It's difficult in the hospital, because it feels like someone is checking on you every hour or so. Nonetheless, sleeping is healing.

Remember that the people who work at the hospital are there to help you feel better. They have difficult jobs. It will be a lovely relief for them to come to your room and see a smile, even if you're in pain. Tell them when you need something and thank them for taking care of you. Refrain from blaming them and try to be grateful for their help. Sometimes this can be challenging, but please don't take it out on the people trying to help you.

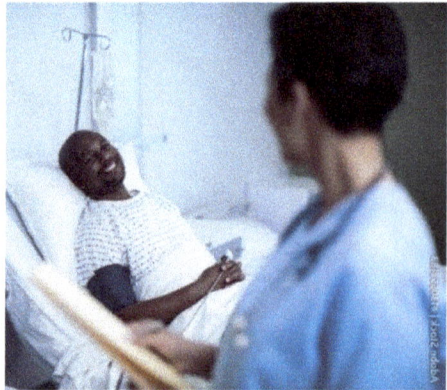

Deep Breathing

Your body has been through trauma, and good deep breathing will help your lungs adjust. Cough and laugh and breathe deeply and slowly. In the hospital, you may have used a spirometer which encourages deep breathing. Continue to use this when you go home. Deep breathing helps you calm your mind and body. Our bodies really like to breathe.

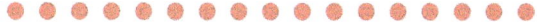

Especially for Spinal Fusion Patients

If you've had a spinal fusion, you have some specific issues for recovery. Your bone graft is healing, forming, and strengthening. Adjacent vertebrae are fusing to one solid bone, and it can take three to 12 months to complete. You'll probably not jump right back into exercising.

During this time, you must be gentle with yourself. Right after your surgery, you'll work with a PT to learn the safest ways to put on and take off your brace, dress, stand, walk, sit, and take part in other activities without putting added stress on your back.

After a few months, when your doctor deems your fusion ready, he will most likely refer you to a physical therapist. The therapist will teach you exercises just for you: what exercises to do, how many, and how often. Pay attention to the form, so you can do it exactly that way each time.

If you suffer with nerve damage, please know that nerves take a long time to heal. It depends on your age, your bones, the damaged location, and your surgery. It could take up to 18 months. Our bodies are amazing, and the nerves will continue to heal, even if it takes longer than we'd like.

Your doctor may recommend a bone growth stimulator after your fusion surgery. It looks something like a fanny pack; you put it around your waist and set the timer. The electrical signals activate the body's natural bone healing process.

Your doctors need to know every prescription and supplement you take. For fusion patients, be sure to check with your doc about supplements, such as anti-inflammatories or fish oil, as they may adversely affect bone graft healing.

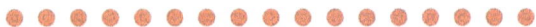

your
first days
at home

Think before you move.

Think before you move.

Think before you move.

Really... stop and think, before you move your body.

For some of us, this is a new idea. Most of our lives are spent without having to think too much about our bodies. Your back, especially these first few days, will demand extra care. Invariably, when one of us falls or wrenches our back, it's because we weren't thinking before we moved. Paying attention can be a hard new habit to create, but your back will thank you for it.

Your doctor will likely tell you:

NO BLTs: No Bending, Lifting, or Twisting.

We would add:

NAPS: No Arching, Pulling, or Straining to Reach.

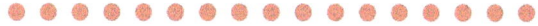

Try to have everything in your world accessible from waist high to shoulder high. Don't reach up to a high cabinet. If something falls on the floor, don't pick it up. Not right now.

During your first few days, please allow yourself to rest and to go slowly. You won't always feel like this, but for right now be "lazy" or "idle." Don't feel guilty for letting your body rest. So many people hate taking time out to rest when their bodies require it. The first days after surgery qualify for required rest. Let your caregivers give you care.

RED LIGHT/GREEN LIGHT

Think before you move, and let pain be your guide. Remember this game you played as a kid? Here's how it will work for you, as you learn how your back feels today:

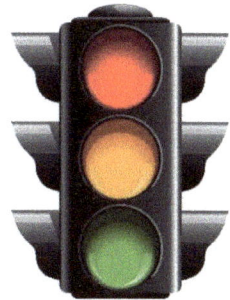

Red Light = STOP = Think = Time Out

This HURTS! Stop whatever you're doing. Take a "time out." Pause. Re-think how you might do this safely. Don't do this today. Try again tomorrow.

Yellow Light = CAUTION = Wait

Pause for a moment and think before you move. Did this hurt last time? You may eventually be able to do this, but maybe not today. Can you do a small part of it? Just a little bit and then a rest? Try that, even though it's difficult for those of us who like to finish a project.

Green Light = Go Gently

Go ahead ... but be mindful as you're moving. Think of how your body feels *right now* and respect that.

your first days at home

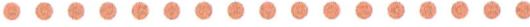

● ● ● ● ● ● ● ● ● ● ● ● ● ● ● ● ● ●

It's natural to be cautious with your back right now, but don't be afraid to move around. Getting up and walking around the house will speed up your recovery, it'll help your digestive system operate properly, and it'll lubricate your joints. It's also pleasant for you to see, smell, hear, and touch something other than your bed or couch.

HOW TO...

Get In and Out of Bed

- Think of yourself as a log, straight, and strong.
- Move your entire torso and thighs together as a single unit.
- Consider wearing satin or silk pajamas. They'll help you slide along the sheets. If the PJs are too warm for you, consider satin or silk sheets. We've even heard of using a trash bag on your bed to help you slide around.

Get Out of Bed

These steps are illustrated on the next page.

- Roll to one side, facing the side you get out on. ❶
- Bring your bottom elbow up under your body. ❷ Use your arms to push up ❸ and bring yourself to a sitting position. ❹
- Stand up slowly and gently.
- Put on your brace. Do this first thing when you get out of bed. Your doctor may recommend putting on your brace while lying down *before* you get up. Whatever doc says, do that.

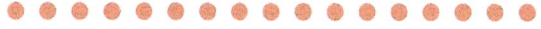

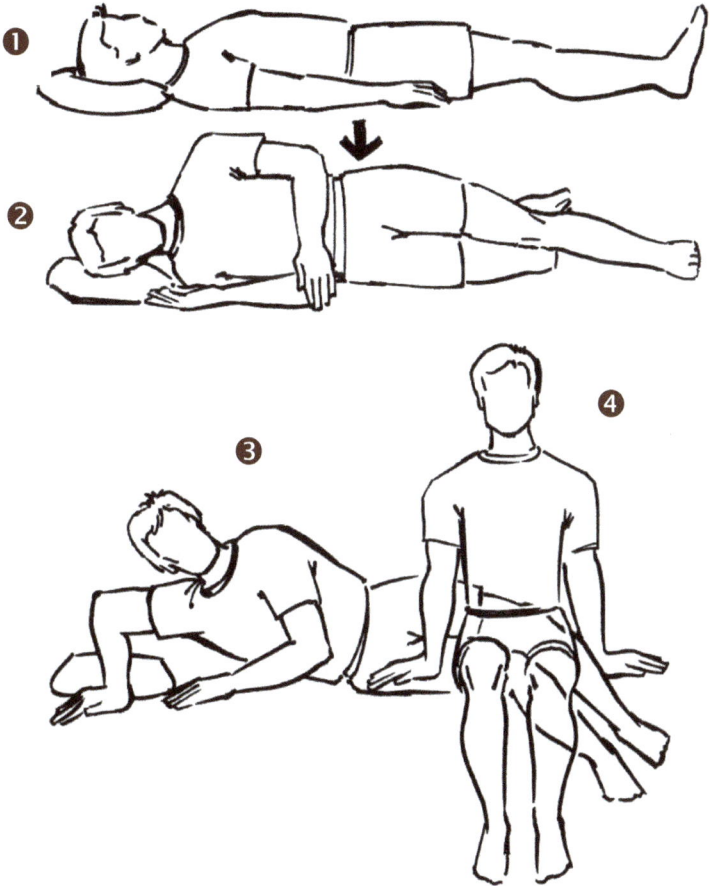

Get Into Bed

- Lower your body gently onto the bed surface.

- Don't "plop" down. This is true for any sitting.

- Visualize yourself using your elbow as a "kickstand" and lean sideways. As you get closer to the bed, bend your knees and bring them up as your torso goes down.

● ● ● ● ● ● ● ● ● ● ● ● ● ● ● ● ● ●

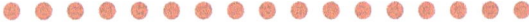

Getting in and out of bed involves the same steps in reverse order, keeping your entire torso (shoulders to hips) straight together and strong.

HOW TO...

Sit Down in a Chair and Get Up from Sitting

- Move slowly and gently. Don't just "plop" down or "jump" up. Hinge at the hips and stick out your butt, lowering yourself until you feel the chair.

- Keep your shoulders and hips aligned. No twisting. If you have to move to the side, think about "pivoting" your entire body rather than twisting your back.

- It's easier to use a chair with a firm seat and with arms, that will help you get down and back up.

- When you're seated, place a small pillow or rolled towel behind your lower back to help you sit up straight. You could also use lumbar support cushions.

- Remember the posture checks from earlier. No slouching! "Don't be a couch, quit the slouch!"

- Before standing, scooch forward to the edge of the chair. That makes it easier to stand up.

- Limit sitting time. Check with your doctor, but after 20-30 minutes of sitting still, you'll need to get up and move around. This amount of time will increase as you get better, but even when you're recovered, you'll want to get up at least once every hour.

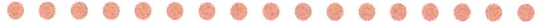

HOW TO...

Get In and Out of a Car

These steps are illustrated below.

- Open the car door, ❶ turn around with your butt facing inside ❷ and sit down. Your feet will remain on the pavement outside the car. Then, one at a time, ❸ swing your legs into the car. ❹

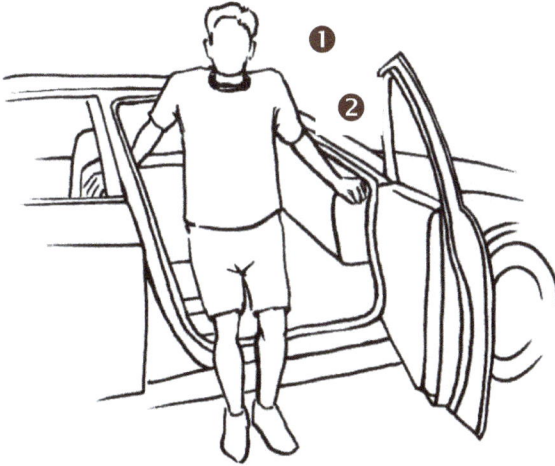

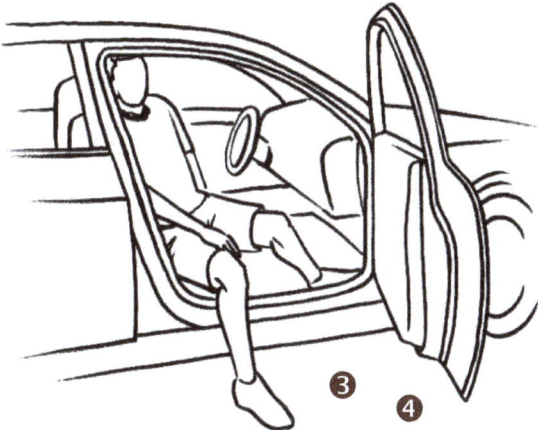

● ● ● ● ● ● ● ● ● ● ● ● ● ● ● ●

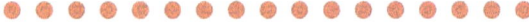

- Do the reverse to get out of the car. Open the car door and swivel your whole body to face the outside. Then, place your feet on the ground in front of you. Once you stand up, take a moment to catch your balance before walking.

- When getting in or out of the car, imagine you're sitting on a Lazy Susan that rotates your entire body. Swivel car seats can be purchased.

- When you're sitting in a car, sit like you're in a chair. Have good posture, keep your feet on the ground, maybe add a support pillow or towel behind you.

- If getting in and out of a car is especially hard for you, consider purchasing a "car door handle" for the inside of the doorframe to support you as you lean on it.

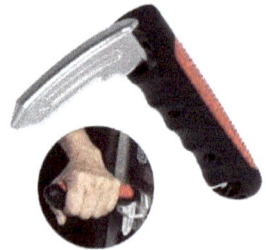

*Car Door Handle
Amazon.com*

HOW TO...

Brush Your Teeth

- Raise items up to your level.

- Don't lean over the sink. Keep standing upright. You may wish to use less water to keep from dribbling.

- Spit into a cup, rather than into the sink.

HOW TO...

Take a Shower

- When turning on the shower, don't lean to pull down the faucet. Instead, use your grabber.

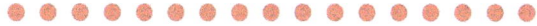

- Consider a shower bench, which can be very helpful for these first few days. Remember, when you pivot, hips and shoulders go together — no twisting.

> It's exhausting for me to wash my hair. Something about holding my hands over my head for so long is hard. I started washing my hair less often, which helps. But my friend Lori suggested that I dip my chin to my chest while I'm shampooing. Such a simple change made the whole process much easier!

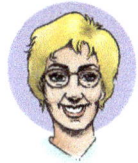

- Guard against raising your arms over your head. It's stressful on the back, so it may be tiring to wash your hair. You don't have to wash your hair every day; at least allow plenty of time for this task. You may try dipping your head forward, chin to chest.

- When you're washing, be sure you remain balanced. You may want to hold onto a handrail or sit on your shower bench.

- Use a bath brush to wash below your knees.

- When you're finished with your shower, sit down to dry off and put on your brace and your clothes.

Wear a cotton t-shirt or camisole underneath your brace. We've found it helpful to prevent sweating or chafing.

- Nix baths or hot tubs for a little while. First, your incision must heal before you immerse it in water. Second, entering and exiting a tub may be difficult right now. Also, you don't want to relax your back muscles while you lie on an angle in the tub.

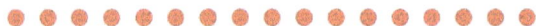

HOW TO...

Reach Up or Down or Across

Remember NAPS — No Arching, Pulling, Stretching!

- Use a grabber for things you cannot reach. You may want to have one in every room, like Lori does!

- Do as little reaching as possible right now. If something drops to the floor, just leave it. Ask a caregiver to pick it up, or to reach a top cabinet for you. It's really best if you don't reach for things during these first few days.

- Putting on shoes and socks can be troublesome right now. Stick with loafers or slippers, or try a long-handled shoehorn or sock aid device.

HOW TO...

Keep Your Bowels Regular

If you take pain medicine, you'll become constipated. After surgery, people often struggle with slowed digestion. Simple measures can prevent or help with constipation. Don't allow your body to go too long without relieving yourself. You should void your bowels at least once every day. Constipation is never fun, but it's worse when your back hurts.

- Drink lots of water/liquid. Eat foods high in fiber.

- Take a fiber supplement or stool softener. Or good old prune juice may just do the trick.

- If you need more help, use MiraLAX®. This gentle laxative can be used every day, which is helpful if you take opioids. It's easier to prevent constipation than to try to fix it. If there's another laxative that your body likes better, please use that.

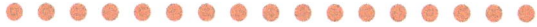

- When sitting on the toilet, don't strain. Let your stomach relax. Don't hold your breath. Try "balloon breathing": purse your lips and blow out. This will engage the muscles that eliminate waste. Gently increase the pressure and sustain it; remember to breathe. Don't bend forward over your legs.

- Allow time and gravity to work. At the same time, don't sit for too long.

- Consider purchasing a Squatty Potty to help with bowel movements. It puts your knees higher than your butt, to help the colon evacuate.

Squatty Potty®

- In general, walking or other gentle exercise will help keep your digestive system working correctly. Yet another good reason to keep moving!

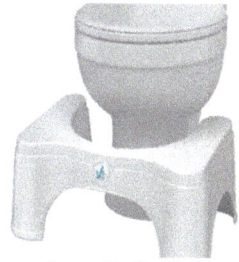

HOW TO...

Put On Makeup or Shave Your Face

- Raise items up to your level. Don't lean down to the countertop.

- Bring a mirror to you, rather than moving your face down or across.

- Be aware of how you're moving your head and neck. When in doubt, move your hand, rather than your head.

HOW TO...

Wear High Heels

- DON'T. Just don't. Seriously. High heels change the curvature of your back and will likely **increase** your back pain.

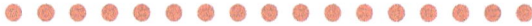

- Wear flat-soled shoes with good arch support, especially in the beginning of your recovery.
- Skip the flip-flops or other open-heeled shoes for now. Stick to sneakers, lace up shoes, flats that have support. You don't want to trip and fall because of your shoes.
- Go barefoot only if it's comfortable for you.
- Please invest in comfortable, supportive, orthopedic shoes. If your feet aren't well supported, then your back will likely suffer. Try orthotic inserts in your current shoes.

Eat Well and Manage Your Weight

Your diet creates the fuel your body needs to heal. Try to eat more healthy foods and fewer processed snacks. Be sure you're getting enough protein, especially now while you're healing. Eat quality proteins, fresh vegetables, fruits, and complex carbs. Getting the right nutrients really will help your recovery. Be sure you're getting enough fiber, even if you're taking a laxative.

What we create in the kitchen is just as important to healthy living as exercise. An effective diet has a variety of foods, with quality proteins, fruits and veggies, and healthy fats.

Being overweight hurts us all in so many ways. Extra weight adds extra pressure especially on your back and knees. It's hard on our bodies to carry added weight. Find a good weight for you and get there. Stay there. Ahhh.... we wish it were just that easy, but it's worth the effort.

There is no magic pill or overnight miracle to help us all lose weight. However, this isn't a weight loss book, so find a plan that works for you. Losing just 10 pounds and keeping it off will make you feel better, look better, and move better!

● ● ● ● ● ● ● ● ● ● ● ● ● ● ● ● ● ●

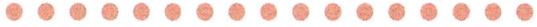

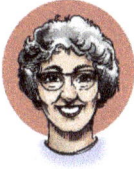

> Weight is a challenge for both of us. When we feel bad, whether from excruciating back pain, or a constant ache, we want to be consoled. Like many people before us, we turn to food for comfort.

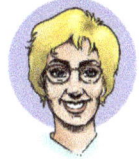

Stay Hydrated

Drink mostly water. Herbal teas are nice. Try to stay away from sodas or energy drinks to reduce caffeine intake and other toxicity. Sugar will increase inflammation, so stay away from that as much as possible. Drinking lots of liquid helps remove toxins built up from the surgery and from being in bed so much.

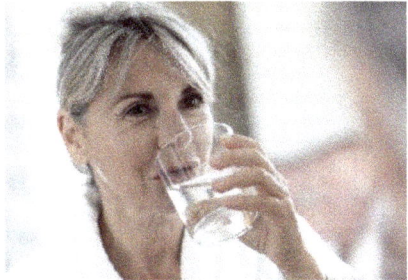

Move Around

You may be tempted to just "stay in bed" all the time, but it's bad for your back. Yes, you need to rest, but you also need to move around when you're awake. Getting up and walking some will help your body heal. Wear your brace and go slowly and gently as you start.

When you've been in one position for an hour, it's time to move around. At least get out of your chair or bed and stretch or walk a little. Stand for a time with your brace on, maybe take the opportunity to go outside or look out the window,

Walking is your primary exercise for these first days of recovery. It reduces pain, aids healing, and prevents blood clots and

● ● ● ● ● ● ● ● ● ● ● ● ● ● ● ●

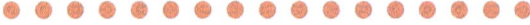

muscle atrophy. Walking boosts blood flow and helps prevent constipation.

Make a "route" inside your home and walk it six or seven times every day. Remember that you cleared paths in your home just for this purpose. Be sure of your footing; don't walk on uneven surfaces. Wear shoes for non-slip assistance. Don't wear just socks on your feet, but barefoot is OK if that feels good to you.

Each day, try to walk a little more. Just a little more.

Rest When You're Tired

Learning to balance between work and rest will be even more important as you get back to your "normal" life. Right now, rest whenever you feel tired. Most of us find that lying flat in bed or on couch is most restful. Find what works best for you. Quality sleep will also help your recovery.

My back really feels better when I lie flat on the floor with my legs up on a chair or couch or ottoman. The 90-degree angle of legs and hips promotes relaxation in my lower back, and our PT says it helps decompress the discs between the vertebrae. Lie in this position for 10-15 minutes.

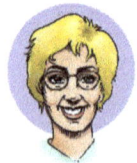

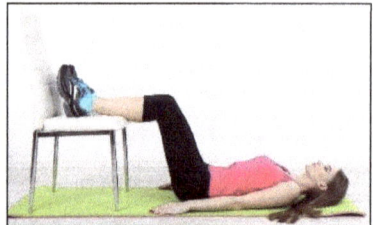

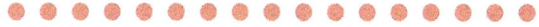

Reduce Anxiety and Stress

We've felt your pain and fear. We know what it's like to hurt so much that you question "Will I ever feel better?" You will… but it will likely take some time. As best you can, try to relax during these first few days. Anxiety, stress, depression, or anger can increase pain. Even muscles can spasm from emotional angst. Stress can aggravate and prolong your pain.

Learn relaxation techniques that work for your body and mind, and do those regularly. Even slowing down your breathing will help. Your friends can support and encourage you. But no one else can do what you need to live well in your body. You have to put in the work.

Reflect on Your Accomplishments

You've been through major surgery. This is an important episode in your life, and it's changed you. Take a few moments each day to reflect. Did something bad happen today? Did you learn something you'll avoid in the future? Did you learn to rest more? Or less? Did something good happen? Celebrate every positive milestone.

After back surgery, no accomplishment is too small to appreciate and celebrate.

- I walked to the mailbox today — woohoo!
- I went to the potty — hurray!
- I took a shower and put on clean clothes — yay!

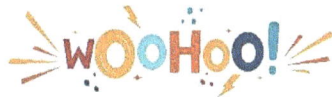

We know it may seem a little silly, but you're worth celebrating!

your first days at home

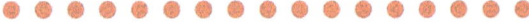

● ● ● ● ● ● ● ● ● ● ● ● ● ● ● ● ● ●

You may consider journaling or writing a blog. Perhaps take a little time each day to think about what's happening with you, your body, your mind, and your spirit. Your life is changed, maybe in ways you haven't understood yet. But life is good, so keep reminding yourself that you're making progress.

After all, taking two steps forward and three steps back is almost like dancing the cha-cha!

Enjoy the dance!

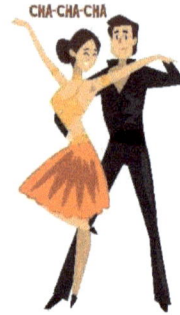

CHA-CHA-CHA

getting
back
to life

RECOVERING FROM SURGERY TAKES TIME

Many of us want to get back to our lives before our backs are ready. Be patient and allow yourself the time it takes to heal. Work your recovery slowly and gradually. Do this by educating yourself about the best ways to keep your back healthy, and then practicing those things regularly. Each body is an amazing vehicle that we need to nurture.

Managing Pain

Keep taking your meds, resting, walking, eating right, and being easy with yourself. Your recovery is not a straight line — you'll have ups and downs.

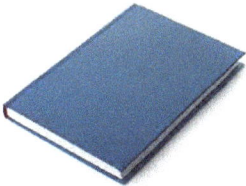

Keeping a pain diary can help you track your progress day by day. It also allows you to look back and see how you're improving.

You'll need to actively manage your pain. Don't wait until you're an "8" before taking medicine. It's easier to prevent pain than to correct pain once it's taken over. Periodically, check in with your back and see what your pain level is right now.

getting back to life

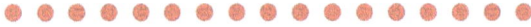

● ● ● ● ● ● ● ● ● ● ● ● ● ● ● ● ●

Is it worse than an hour ago? Is it better? Do you expect it to be worse in the next hour? This is a good time to make a note in your pain diary.

> Sitting is especially painful for me, yet I need to spend two or three hours each day working at my computer. So, I know that my pain will get worse while I'm working. Rather than waiting for it, I take pain meds at the beginning of my computer session. By anticipating my need, I use less medicine to relieve my pain while causing less trauma to my body. I also get up at least once every hour to move around, like every good back patient should!

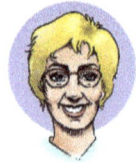

Follow-up Is the Key to Your Recovery

The quality of your recovery is better when you incorporate proper movement and exercise into your life. Your PT has taught you exercises, how to do them, for how long, and how often. Now it's your responsibility to do them regularly at home. These are the basis of your new healthy life. You're taking charge of your own health.

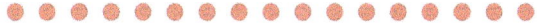

We each have exercises that we're supposed to do daily. Some days, we just don't want to... (Have you had days like that?) Whenever we complain that our backs hurt, we ask ourselves "Why didn't we do our exercises?" Usually we've neglected them, and our backs complain!

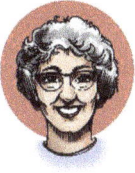

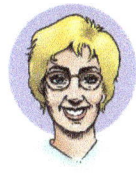

FIND EXERCISE YOU'LL ACTUALLY DO

Your back will not thrive with a sedentary lifestyle. Staying active is one of the best things you can do for yourself. When your doc gives you the OK, it's time to find an exercise program that you'll enjoy and continue for the rest of your life. It may be a workout at your gym, or walking, or riding a bike. It doesn't have to be complicated, but it does need to be regular.

This is a good time to try out new exercises. When you start something new, remember your new habit of thinking before you move. If you're taking a class, speak to the teacher first and find out what modifications you can make. As a general rule: if it hurts, don't do it. Start slowly and gently, especially for your first class. If that goes well, then you can do more during the next class. The more you exercise, the more you can move confidently and strongly.

Listen to your body while you're exercising.

● ● ● ● ● ● ● ● ● ● ● ● ● ● ● ● ● ● ●

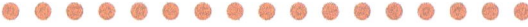

The fitness concept of "No Pain No Gain" is a BIG LIE.

We're adamant about eliminating "No Pain No Gain."
Let's avoid a "push past your pain limit" mentality. If an
exercise hurts, don't do it. Pain is your
body's way of saying "not right now."
Listen to what your body is telling you.
Sometimes an exercise will stretch you or
make you sore, which is an uncomfortable
feeling that stops after a short time.

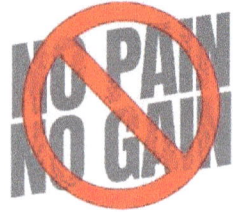

*Pain that doesn't abate should never be a part of your
workout. Exercise should make you feel better, not worse!*

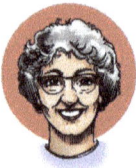

Neither of us are exercisers by nature, but
we've each learned to love our
workouts. They improve mood and
stress levels. Endorphins created by
exercise reduce pain and help us feel
better overall. Heart and lung functions
improve, as well as circulation. Exercise also
helps keep our weight down, which is another
important part of this new life.

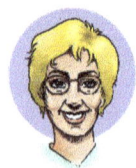

Walking

Walking is a good, low-impact exercise for your whole body,
and especially your back. When you're in pain, you tend to
shuffle your feet. Have you noticed that? Instead, pick up your
feet, keep your head level, looking forward, shoulders back
and down. Stride evenly heel-toe, heel-toe, pushing off with
your big toe. Swing your arms naturally.

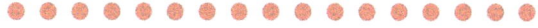

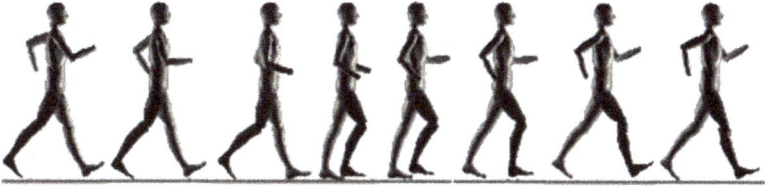

Start out slowly and walk for a short time. Start really small — try just two or three minutes. Remember that when you walk three minutes, you'll have to walk three minutes back. After a few days of three minutes, try five minutes out and back. Or try three minutes twice a day, or maybe three times tomorrow. Build up gradually.

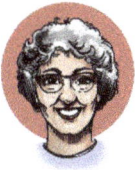

> After each of my surgeries, I would increase my walking by going to Costco. I like the open space, the buggy handles are high enough that I have to stand up straight, and it feels like I can walk forever!

Water Exercise

Working out or just walking in the water reduces the load on your joints, and you get relief from gravity with the buoyancy of water. You can strengthen and relax muscles and improve your mobility more safely in the water.

If you're a good swimmer, then swim laps. Swim just 5 minutes to start. We recommend free style and back stroke. These are gentle styles of swimming that don't arch or twist your back. As always, check with your doctor first.

● ● ● ● ● ● ● ● ● ● ● ● ● ● ● ● ● ● ●

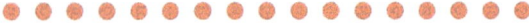

Yoga, Tai Chi, and Pilates

Yoga, Tai Chi, and Pilates are great strength and balance builders. If you're just starting out, try a class for senior citizens; you don't have to be a senior to attend, but those classes will be gentler. Find classes that you and your body love. The scheduled routine makes it easier to work out regularly.

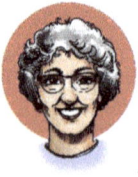

> I've recently discovered Pilates, and I love it! It tones, strengthens, and lengthens my muscles and my body. I walk away feeling taller! Pilates is all about my core, and flexibility, and helping my balance. It has given me better stability, coordination, and endurance.

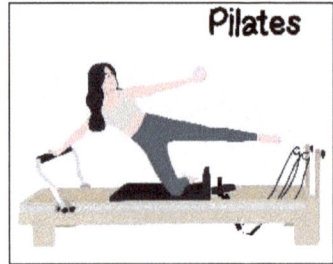

Pilates

Strength Training

Whether you lift weights or use your bodyweight, strength training is essential. Your PT can show you which moves are best for you and your back. For good posture and less back pain, build up strength in your:

- **Core.** Remember that core is not just your abdomen, it's your front, back, and sides. We're not interested in a "six-pack of abs." We all want strength and health for good balance and to walk and move well.

- **Back.** At first, it may feel uncomfortable strengthening your back. These are big muscles that need to be strong to support your vertebrae and correct posture.

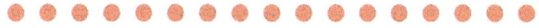

- **Buttocks.** These are the largest muscles in the body for a reason! These muscles help you stay upright and keep your body moving forward. Gluteus maximus, medias and minimus work together for leg movement. Strong gluteals are important for pelvic alignment and walking.

- **Hips.** They are the hinges on which your body moves. Strengthen hips and thigh muscles also for sideways motion, inside and outside of your thighs.

- **Pelvic floor.** This muscular sling across the base of your pelvis supports bowel, bladder, and reproductive organs. The muscles and nerves from your back are directly connected to those in the pelvic floor. As we age, the pelvic muscles are often overlooked, and they can cause pain that feels like back pain. We all want to avoid pelvic problems like leakage or losing control of bowel or bladder. If you're having trouble in this area, please see your doctor or ask for a referral for pelvic physical therapy.

  A good pelvic floor exercise is Kegels, which can benefit both men and women. There are many resources to learn about Kegels, but here's a quick version: pretend you're stopping your urine stream. Squeeze those muscles while standing, sitting, walking, reclining, in bed, in all different positions. Do these as often as you can remember — four to five times a day.

- **Legs, knees, ankles, feet.** Good posture and strong bodies start at the bottom. It seems like feet and ankles are left out of regular exercise regimens. We've found it very important to strengthen and work our feet. If your feet or your walking gait is off-kilter, then the rest of your body is out of alignment. A strong lower body also helps with balance. Try some good orthotic shoes or inserts to improve your overall posture.

getting back to life

● ● ● ● ● ● ● ● ● ● ● ● ● ● ● ● ●

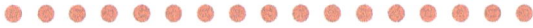

LEARN PROPER BODY MECHANICS

For us, the biggest change was to stop and think before we move. That's why we've stressed it so much in this book. Many people live on autopilot, not considering their bodies. Now you need to think about how each movement will affect your back before you move. Soon it will become a habit, and you won't have to stop and think so often.

Sitting

Good sitting posture starts with your feet flat on the ground. Don't cross your legs because it twists your spine. Seriously, don't cross your legs anymore. Knees should be just below the height of your hips.

Be centered in your chair, not leaning to one side, or forward or backward. Let your back touch the back of your chair. You can place a pillow or lumbar cushion behind you to help maintain good posture and a straighter spine. When you sit, your circulation suffers. Postural cushions promote good blood flow to your legs. Keep your shoulders down and back, and gently lift the top of your skull to lengthen your neckline.

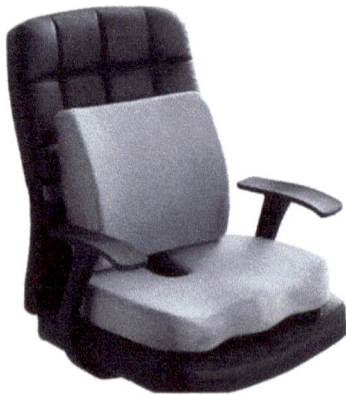

Remember to get up at least once every hour. Don't remain sedentary for long periods. It's bad for your back, your heart, and your circulatory system. If you've sat for a while, you'll probably be stiff when you stand up. Take a moment to pause and gather your balance before walking away.

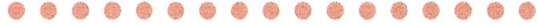

When you're sitting in front of a computer, be sure that the position of your desk and chair are ergonomically correct. The keyboard and mouse should be around chair arm height. Monitor should be slightly lower than eyesight. Generally, if you look straight ahead, you should be looking at the top of your monitor. Looking slightly down at your screen will help with posture and neck or shoulder pain. Consider adjusting your monitor up and down regularly to keep your head at different angles.

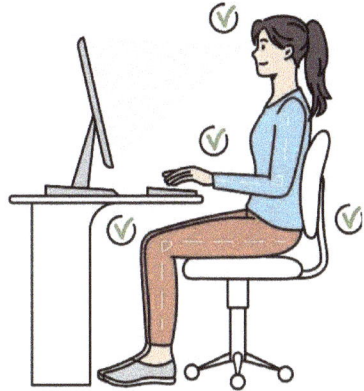

Standing

Good standing posture will mean less back pain.

- Keep your feet solidly on the floor, about hip width apart.
- Balance your weight through heels, arches, and toes.
- Don't shift your weight from side to side or front to back.
- Keep your knees soft: not locked, straight but relaxed.
- Gently draw in your lower abdomen; think of sucking in your belly button to your spine.
- Engage the muscles of your pelvic floor with Kegels.
- Gently draw your shoulders back and down, lift the top of your skull. Think tall. Imagine a string running from the bottom of your spine through the top of your head and pulling gently upward.

This is probably very different from what you're accustomed to, and it will take time for your body to learn these better habits.

●●●●●●●●●●●●●●●●●●

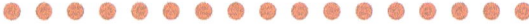

When standing for a long time, you can ease your back pain by placing one foot on a higher surface.

- While standing for a while (for instance, in the grocery checkout line), relieve yourself temporarily by placing one foot on lowest rung of the shopping cart. Even leaning your elbows on the shopping cart handle can give your back some temporary relief. Don't stay there for too long; hunched over is not good posture.

- If you're washing dishes, open the cabinet beneath the sink, and place one foot on the cabinet floor. Change feet from time to time.

- Lean on a countertop or desk. It's just a temporary relief, but it still feels good.

- Try just lifting one heel; that releases some of the pressure on your back.

Lifting and Carrying

Your doctor should tell you how much you can lift. Most recommend no more than 10 pounds. A gallon of water weighs a little over eight pounds, so does a small cat. You'll be able to lift more as you recover and regain your strength. When you're carrying anything, keep it close to your body. Hug it if you can. Ask your PT for techniques specific for you. Remember to lift with your legs, not your back.

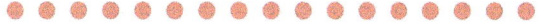

Reaching Down to the Floor

- Bend your knees every time you reach, especially reaching down. This will help protect your back from arching.

- Keep both feet on the floor, with both knees bent.

- When reaching down, try to have something nearby to hold onto, so that you don't lose your balance.

- Try the **Golfer's Lift** (illustrated below). Notice that he's placing his hands on a steady surface nearby. Then, bend the knee that bears weight. The other leg can be behind you for counterbalance.

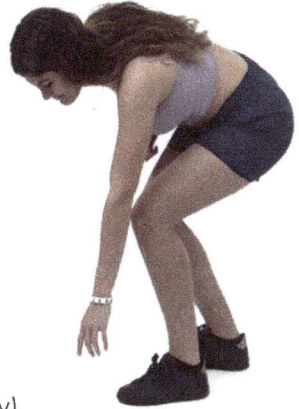

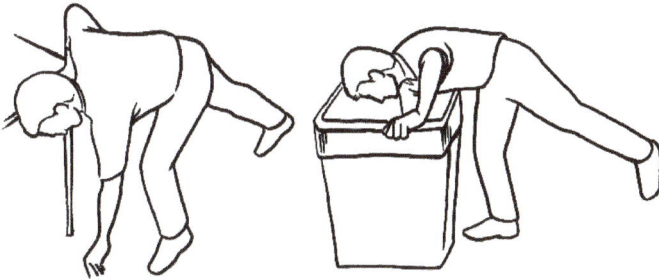

Having Sex

Generally, sex is a healthy activity for back patients. It's pleasurable, it boosts circulation, and it produces endorphins that help reduce pain. Ask your doc when you can resume sexual activities.

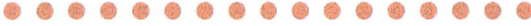

getting back to life

● ● ● ● ● ● ● ● ● ● ● ● ● ● ● ● ● ●

Driving

Think of the seat of your car as a chair. Use lumbar support for the curve of your back and press your back into the seat. It's best if your knees are lower than your hips. Raise the seat if possible and be sure you can see over the steering wheel. Adjust your steering wheel to what feels right for you, up and down, as well as closer and further. Adjust the headrest for your comfort and safety.

Remember the right way to get in and out of your car (see page 59). If you drive for longer than an hour, plan a rest stop. Get out and stretch or walk a little.

Please remember that you shouldn't drive while taking painkillers. Your reaction times will be slower, and you may not be safe.

Falling

We've talked about preventing a fall, but what happens when you do fall? *It's unlikely you'll have time to find and read this book as you're falling, so here are some tips for your brain to remember while it's happening.*

- Stay loose. Try not to tense up. Relaxed bodies are less likely to be seriously injured.
- Breathe as you fall and keep breathing.
- Bend your arms and legs as you're falling. Try not to "catch yourself" with your hands, as you will likely injure your wrists.
- Protect your head, tucking chin down and lowering your head, perhaps covering your head with your arms or hands.

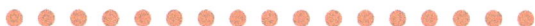

- If you're falling face down, do your best to turn your entire body to the side, not twisting your back, but turning to fall onto your side. At the very least, try to turn your face to the side, protecting your head.

- Roll on impact, as best you can.

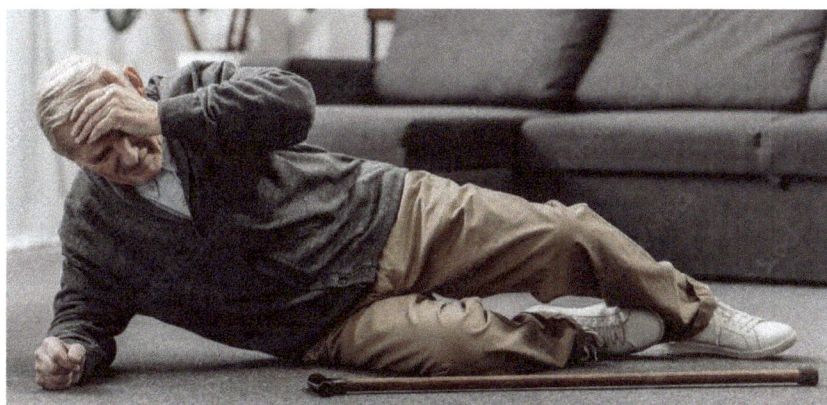

Getting Up from the Floor

Whether you've fallen to the floor or purposefully sat down on the floor, get back up without straining your back.

- After you've fallen, try not to panic. Pause for a moment and breathe and assess your situation. Scan your body for injuries. Get your bearings. There's no need to hurry back up, so take your time.

- If it's safe to move around, roll onto your side. Then, remembering the technique for getting out of bed (see page 56), roll over onto your hands and knees.

- Crawl on your hands and knees to the nearest stable piece of furniture: chair, sofa, table, counter. Place a hand, or both hands if you prefer, steady on the piece of furniture.

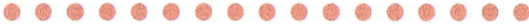

- Keep your back rounded to protect it. Move your strongest leg, putting your foot flat on the floor. You're now in a one-legged kneeling position.

- Move your other foot to the floor so you're almost standing, still holding onto the piece of furniture, still rounding your back.

- If you're next to a chair, then slowly turn around and sit. If not, then roll your back up to standing, starting with your knees bent, then hips under, then rolling up one vertebra at a time.

RE-THINK REGULAR ACTIVITIES

Everyday movements can cause pain if they're done without consideration for your back. We all must figure out how to accomplish those tasks without adding to our pain. You'll take what you've learned already and apply it to any task or activity. For instance, house cleaning is hard work and can increase back pain. Here are some ideas for making cleaning easier on your back.

General House Cleaning Chores

- Can someone else do these tasks for you? That would be awesome!

- Try working for a short time (5 minutes) and see how you feel. Clean in stages. Do a little now, a little later, and finish tomorrow! You don't have to do it all at once.

- Consider your body position while you're doing the activity. Keep your knees bent, pull in your belly button (which engages your core), don't twist.

- Remember that no one is coming to your home to inspect with white gloves. Try to lower your stress about what your home "should" look like.

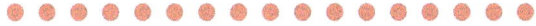

Vacuuming

- Can you get a lighter-weight vacuum cleaner, or a robot vacuum?
- Make the "push and pull" movements of vacuuming smaller so that you're not reaching and bending so much.
- Do one room and then rest.

Sweeping & Mopping

- Like vacuuming, make your "push and pull" movements smaller.
- Try using a Swiffer® instead of a heavy mop.
- Try using a steam mop, where you only push (without pulling).

Loading & Emptying the Dishwasher or Washing Machine

- Bend your knees before bending down.
- Use a grabber rather than your hands.
- Create smaller loads so that there's not so much to handle at once.

Consider other activities you do regularly and rearrange your movements to keep your back happy!

Making the bed

Laundry

Dishes

Cleaning

Taking a shower

Cooking

Leaving home

Staying organized

Getting dressed

Grocery shopping

Keeping plants alive

Travelling

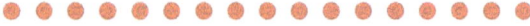

● ● ● ● ● ● ● ● ● ● ● ● ● ● ● ● ●

OVERDOING

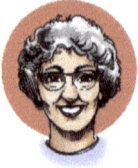

We both are natural over-doers. There are times we make plans without thinking whether our bodies are up to the task. In fact, the overwhelming majority of back-pain sufferers we've met over many years do the same. We're all high achievers, people who give 110%. We're ambitious and motivated to do more, have more, be more. But now, we're pretty sure that this attitude has had a negative effect on our bodies and the causes of our pain.

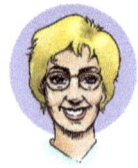

As you continue to recover, we recommend that you reconsider your habits, your patterns of living, and the activities and mindsets that are no longer helpful. Learn to say "no," to prioritize self-care, and to practice resting your body and your mind.

When you find yourself overdoing... with the weekend sports friends who call you to be in the game... or the long-term project that requires late nights at the office... or with the kids who want you to play tag with them... if you've overdone, then your body may have more pain in the next few days.

The "necessary down time" for overdoing can take you by surprise, or you can plan for it. Try to anticipate when you'll overdo, and you can plan extra down time before and afterwards.

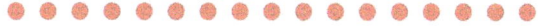

MIND BODY CONNECTION

Feeling Down in the Dumps?

Ohhh…. you're having a bad day! And you're in the dumps. Yuck! All of us feel this way from time to time, and it's OK! You're allowed to feel whatever emotions come up: angry, betrayed, disappointed, hopeless, powerless, sad, grieving… you need to feel your feelings. Here's the key – go ahead and have a pity party, just DON'T STAY THERE!

Remember that you are in charge of your health, and you can control what your brain thinks.

How to Lift Yourself out of the Dumps

- **Be mindful.** The idea behind mindfulness is that you put away the worry. You don't stress or even dream about the future or the past. You're right here, right now. You simply notice your thoughts and feelings, all without judgment. Mindfulness works best if you practice it each day.

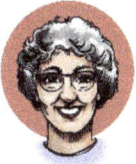

Being present and quieting my mind helps me stay balanced. Taking a moment to pause, slowing down my breath, is grounding for me.

- **Try mindful activities.** Like meditation, yoga, and tai chi, these routines help you step back from the constant thoughts that run through your brain. This turns out to be a powerful way to change your perspective on life and gain more control over your ups and downs.

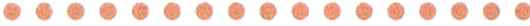

- **Simplify your life.** If your life feels jam-packed with work and chores, it can be hard to remember you have an inner self. Slow down. Cut out what you can. Sometimes, you need to tell yourself "It's OK to do less" or just stop altogether.

- **Express yourself.** Art can be a healthy and safe creative way to voice your feelings. It's not hard to get started. Find a hobby you love, an old one or a new one. The results don't matter. Push past your doubts and give artistic expression a shot. You may find that you enjoy it much more than you expect. Here are some ideas:

  - **Write.** The very act of writing can help your brain. Try journaling, or just writing whatever comes to mind.

  - **Doodle.** Grab some colored pencils, or a coloring book, or just a blank piece of paper. Find a quiet spot and draw away.

  - **Music.** Listening to music is very calming to the soul.

  - **New hobbies.** Experiment to see what you might like.

- **Have fun.** Make fun a priority. Your inner self needs some serious outer fun. Do something that makes you happy. Keep at it. You'll be lifted in no time.

  - Swing in the park.

  - Go somewhere you love.

  - Sing along to your radio in the car.

  - Watch a funny video.

  - Laugh with a friend… preferably laugh until you are gasping for breath!

- **Call a "time out."** Just as if you were a little kid, sometimes you need a break to get a better handle on situations. So, when you're overwhelmed, don't be afraid to call a "time out" for yourself. Do something

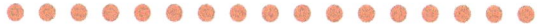

relaxing, even set up times during the day that you can consciously relax and stick to that routine.

- **Watch the negative self-talk.** That voice in your head isn't really you. It's often trying to sabotage your feelings, and you can learn to ignore it. It's not easy, but please don't beat yourself up. You're doing the best you can, and that's enough.

- **Find a purpose.** When your life lacks purpose, you feel lost and you don't have any direction. When you feel a strong sense of purpose, you tend to be more skilled at working through life's challenges. Purpose can come through spirituality, through your job, through volunteer work. It doesn't have to be your "ultimate life's purpose" – it's enough to give you purpose right now.

- **Help someone else.** When you reach out past your own pain to help another person, your perspective will re-align, and you'll remember your problems aren't so bad after all.

I learn from the people I teach in the pool. At first their pain is so overwhelming that they can only see themselves. As they get to know other people in pain, and move around more, and start to feel better – they will begin to see other people's needs. I love seeing this progress, because it means that they're healing and seeing beyond their own problems.

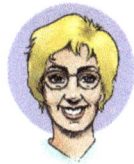

- **Give thanks.** When you focus on things you're grateful for, it lifts you up. It shifts your thoughts and helps you focus on what's positive in your life.

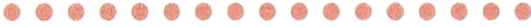

- **Smile.** Smile inwardly to let your body know that all is well. When you smile outwardly, it's good for you and for the world around you.

Relaxation

Relaxation doesn't mean you're doing nothing or being lazy. Think of it as a necessity, like the other necessities of life. Like proper eating and sleeping, relaxing helps to keep you well.

Relaxation skills are a great way to help with stress management. Decreasing the stress on your mind and body can help you cope with everyday stress, long-term stress, and stress related to pain.

Some benefits of relaxation:

- It slows your heart and breathing rate, lowers your blood pressure, controls blood sugar levels, increases blood flow, reduces muscle tension.
- It improves focus, mood, and sleep.
- It helps reduce pain and fatigue.

Practice. Be patient with yourself.
Don't let these efforts become yet another stressor!

Learning How to Relax

This one is often overlooked, but a body that holds stress tends to be a body in pain. Learning how to calm your body and mind can help you keep your pain under control.

For instance, sprinkle your day with short activities, like taking a walk for just few minutes. Rather than one long routine, these little walks can keep stress at bay and ease tension levels throughout your day.

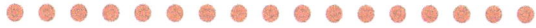

There are many ways to relax, and we encourage you to try out several to find which can work for you. Here is an easy one that you can do any time and any place: breathing.

- Count how long you breathe in and how long you breathe out. This is your starting point.

- Now, try to breathe out a little longer than you're breathing in. For instance, if your starting point was "in for 2, out for 2," then breathe out for 3. Do that a couple of times. Then breathe out for 4. Continue until you're breathing out twice as long as you're breathing in. "In for 2, our for 4" is an example.

- Now, try to breathe in for a little longer. With our example, now breathe "in for 3, out for 4." Do that a couple of times. Then, breathe out for 5. Then breathe out for 6. Continue that.

- A good goal for slow, relaxed breathing is "in for 4, out for 8." Some people like a hold in between, like "in for 4, hold for 4, out for 8." Try variations to see which numbers of relaxed breathing feel best for you.

Remember, we're making life changes. You don't have to make big changes, but consistency is your goal. We're re-aligning our bodies and our minds for less pain.

As we leave you, we want to remind you that there is a way back from chronic back pain, either with or without surgery. We have given you support, information, and education to aid in your recovery. Don't let stress and pain overwhelm you. Recovery and relief take time. Use all the modalities you have available to give you your best outcome.

● ● ● ● ● ● ● ● ● ● ● ● ● ● ● ● ● ● ●

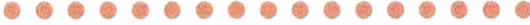

WEBSITES WE USE REGULARLY

When you're researching on the internet, please don't believe everything you read. Check that your sources are reputable. Blogs can be helpful for people documenting their own journeys, but their situations may not match up with your reality.

Here are some sites that we use for ourselves.

For medical expertise and scientific information:

- **WebMD**, *WebMD.com*

- **Cleveland Clinic**, *My.ClevelandClinic.org/Health*

- **Johns Hopkins Health Info**, *HopkinsMedicine.org/Health*

- **Nutrition and Supplement** information with scientific support, *Examine.com*

For living with back pain:

- **But You Don't Look Sick** is great for "invisible" pain. Check out the "Spoon Theory" to explain fatigue to your loved ones, *ButYouDontLookSick.com*

- **The Better Way Back** is no longer updated, but still has great info, *TheBetterWayBack.org*

- **Mindfulness** for learning how to calm your mind and be more 'present,' *Mindful.org*

www.ingramcontent.com/pod-product-compliance
Lightning Source LLC
Chambersburg PA
CBHW052024030426

42335CB00026B/3269